P9-DNB-195

Erratum:

The last line of text on page 57 should appear
as the first line of text on page 60.

GROWING
YOUNG

Other titles by Ashley Montagu:

ON BEING HUMAN
MAN'S MOST DANGEROUS MYTH: *The Fallacy of Race*
DARWIN, COMPETITION, AND COOPERATION
THE NATURAL SUPERIORITY OF WOMEN
IMMORTALITY
PRENATAL INFLUENCES
MAN IN PROCESS
THE HUMANIZATION OF MAN
THE DOLPHIN IN HISTORY
MAN'S EVOLUTION
THE IDEA OF RACE
THE HUMAN REVOLUTION
THE ANATOMY OF SWEARING
SEX, MAN AND SOCIETY
THE IGNORANCE OF CERTAINTY
TOUCHING
THE ELEPHANT MAN
THE NATURE OF HUMAN AGGRESSION
HUMAN EVOLUTION

GROWING YOUNG

—— by ——
Ashley Montagu

*In our innermost soul we are children
and remain so for the rest of our lives.*
—SIGMUND FREUD

McGRAW-HILL BOOK COMPANY
New York   St. Louis   San Francisco   Toronto

1 2 3 4 5 6 7 8 9 0 D O D O 8 7 6 5 4 3 2 1

LIBRARY OF CONGRESS CATALOGING IN PUBLICATION DATA

Montague, Ashley, 1905–
Growing young.
Includes bibliographical references.
1. Youthfulness. 2. Rejuvenation. I. Title.
BF724.M64   155   81-8433
ISBN 0-07-042841-7   AACR2

Book design by Stanley S. Drate

Dedicated to
Preston Tuttle

Contents

Preface

Sometimes one has to say difficult things,
but one has to say them as simply as possible.
—G. P. HARDY
A Mathematician's Apology

This book represents the result of many years of work and study in a large variety of fields, seemingly unrelated, but actually all bearing upon the better understanding of the nature of human nature, and the significance of that understanding for the healthy development of the person and of humanity. It is essentially a book of discovery, really an adventure story, but one which is solidly based on the research findings of innumerable scientists and thinkers. The ideas presented in this book involve a whole new way of thinking about human beings, which should be part of the mental equipment of everyone. But that the reader will be able to decide for himself.

Here I should like to thank the many kind people who read the book in manuscript and gave me much help in making this a better book than it would otherwise have been. These are Weston La Barre, Emeritus Professor of Anthropology at Duke University; Dr. Robert Butler, Director of the National Institute of Aging; Dr. Thomas J. Cottle; Dr. Judith Economos; Renate Fernandez; Suzanne Fremon; Drs. Philip and Julia Gordon; Professor Roderic Gorney, Department of Psychiatry, University of California at Los Angeles; Professor Stephen Jay Gould, Museum

ix

of Comparative Zoology, Harvard University; Dr. Judith Lynne Hanna; Professor Floyd Matson, Department of American Studies, University of Hawaii at Honolulu; and Preston Tuttle.

I also thank Helen Zimmerberg, Louise Schaeffer, and Elizabeth Hynes of the Biology Library, and Terry Caton, Janice Welburn, and Pat Swift of the Psychology Library, at Princeton University, also Louise Yorke of the Library at Princeton Medical Center, for all their courtesies and assistance. And finally, to McGraw-Hill Senior Editor Gladys Justin Carr and her assistant editor Leslie Meredith, I am indebted for their always gracious help.

Princeton, New Jersey   ASHLEY MONTAGU

Communication
from a
Flying Saucer

The trouble with earthlings is their early adulthood. As long as they are young, they are lovable, open-hearted, tolerant, eager to learn and to collaborate. They can even be induced to play with one another. Most adults, however, are mortal enemies. The only educational problem earth has is how to keep them young.

For life, evolution, progress, and adaptation to new situations they are useful only as long as they keep their youthful qualities. But the funny thing is that in all the educational institutions I visited the object was to hasten maturity instead of delaying it. Surely your history can teach you that only the races with the longest childhood were able to remain in the cultural mainstream. The ideal should be to prolong childhood up to sixty years. Then you would be able to produce a real planetary culture.

Once you realize the importance of this prolongation it will be easy for your biologists to work out the necessary techniques to keep your children teachable. Your cultural life has already become too rich, too complicated, for you to content yourselves with an educational period of a mere twelve years. True specialization should start at sixty.

Compare the growth of intelligence in human children of, let us say, seven to fourteen, with that of children of fourteen to twenty-one. Do you see the dramatic slowdown the moment maturity appears? Many children simply stop at sixteen, some even at fourteen. And even those who go on evolving usually progress along lines already laid down at the age of ten or twelve. No new regions of mind normally open in human beings after that.

"The most shocking fact about evolution is not that we descend from something we probably wouldn't like to meet alone in a forest at night, but that something descends from us which we certainly wouldn't like to meet even at noon in a crowded street. Perhaps the subhuman is more acceptable than the suprahuman.'

Equals One, 1969–2   *The Journal of Auroville,*
                                                Pondicherry 2, India

Introduction

Childhood is the name of the world's immediate
future; of such, and such alone, is the promise of the
kingdom of man.
                                    —WALTER DE LA MARE
                                      Early One Morning

Growing young, the title and the subject of this book, is a process that has played a fundamental role in the evolution of the
human species and in the development of every human being
who has ever lived. Moreover, its significance and its ramifications for the future of each of us and of humanity in general are
so staggering that an understanding of it should be a part of
everyone's equipment. Yet as a scientific principle it is known
only to a few scientists; others—the vast numbers of human
beings whose lives might be changed by the application of this
principle—are ignorant of it. To fill that void, to explain the
meaning of "growing young," is the purpose of this book.

The process of growing young is known as *neoteny* or
paedomorphosis. These terms, which will be explained in detail in
the following pages and in the appendix on the history of the
concept, refer to the retention into adult life of those human
traits associated with childhood, with fetuses, and even with the
juvenile and fetal traits of our primitive ancestors. Neoteny is
also used to refer to the slowing down of the rate of development
and the extension of the phases of development from birth to
old age.

I

This is a concept that is not easy to understand. We see evidence before us all the time that adults are different from children, and we think we know that an adult human being is nothing like the fetus curled up in his mother's womb. Furthermore, we tend to believe that this is the way things should be: "Grown-ups" and children are two separate classes of beings, and because adults possess the power and the strength, we spend the years of our childhood yearning to be grown up. Many of us in our youth falsified our ages in an effort to seem older than we really were. And as we approached the end of schooling and the beginning of what we were taught was "real" life, we rejoiced that we were finally becoming adults and different from children.

Yet the truth about the human species is that in body, spirit, feeling, and conduct we are designed to grow and develop in ways that emphasize rather than minimize childlike traits. We are intended to remain in many ways childlike; we were never intended to grow "up" into the kind of adults most of us have become.

It is the purpose of this book to show how the principle of neoteny has affected first our physical evolution and development, and then the evolution of our behavior. Finally, we will see that the role it is designed to play in our social development is of fundamental significance. We will realize that the retention of juvenile physical traits is one of the major qualities that differentiate human beings from other animals, and that when this quality is carried over from physical traits to behavioral patterns, human beings can revolutionize their lives and become for the first time, perhaps, the kinds of creatures their heritage intends them to be—that is, youthful all the days of our lives.

What, precisely, are those traits of childhood behavior that are so valuable and that tend to disappear gradually as human beings grow older? We have only to watch children to see them clearly displayed: Curiosity is one of the most important; imaginativeness; playfulness; open-mindedness; willingness to experiment; flexibility; humor; energy; receptiveness to new ideas; honesty; eagerness to learn; and perhaps the most pervasive and the most valuable of all, the need to love. All normal children, unless they have been corrupted by their elders, show these qualities every day of their childhood years. They ask questions endlessly:

"Why?" "What is it?" "What's it for?" "How does it work?"
They watch and they listen. They want to know everything about
everything. They can keep themselves busy for hours with the
simplest toys, endowing sticks and stones and featureless objects
with personalities and histories, imagining elaborate stories
about them, building sagas that continue day after day, month
after month. They play games endlessly, sometimes carefully
constructing the rules, sometimes developing the game as they
go along. They accept changes without defensiveness. When
they try to accomplish something and fail, they are able to try to
do it another way, and another, until they find that it works.
They laugh—babies learn to smile and laugh before they can
even babble—and children laugh from sheer exuberance and
happiness. Unless they suspect they may be punished for it, they
tell the truth; they call the shots as they see them. And they soak
up knowledge and information like sponges; they are learning all
the time; every moment is filled with learning.

How many adults retain these qualities into middle age? Few.
They tend to stop asking those questions that will elicit information. Not many adults, when confronted with something unfamiliar, ask as children always do, "What is it?" "What is it for?"
"Why?" "How does it work?" Most adults draw back from the
unfamiliar, perhaps because they are reluctant to demonstrate
ignorance, perhaps because they have become genuinely indifferent to the interesting experiences of life and consider that
absorbing something new into the old patterns is simply too
much trouble.

Nor can most adults content themselves with simple play-
things enriched by the imagination. Witness the enormous
growth of industries that cater to the "leisure-time" and "recre-
ational" activities of adults, that manufacture the toys that
grown-ups need in order to play: boats, cars, trailers, equipment
for camping and hiking and running and tennis and golf, television sets, movies, sporting events, equipment for travel and even
for shopping. The list seems endless. This is not to say, of
course, that these activities are not enjoyable and healthful, but
it is to say that most of them are elaborate beyond the dreams of
children. The difference, it has been said, between the men and
the boys is the price of the toys. Very few adults in our affluent

Western civilization are able to maintain themselves by themselves, with the help only of their imaginations and their own
physical energies. They need to bolster their efforts with huge
amounts of expensive equipment. ⚹

Most adults have lost, too, the ability to laugh from sheer
happiness; perhaps they have lost happiness itself. In any case,
adulthood as we know it brings sobriety and seriousness along
with its responsibilities. Most adults have also lost their ability to
tell the simple truth; many appear to have lost the ability to
discern a simple truth in the complex morass they live in.

Perhaps the saddest loss of all is the gradual erosion of the
eagerness to learn. Most adults stop any conscious effort to learn
early in their adulthood, and never thereafter actively pursue
knowledge or understanding in any form. It is as though they
believed that they had learned all they needed to know, and
understood it all, and had found the best possible attitudes toward it, by the age of eighteen or twenty-two or whenever they
stopped their formal schooling. At this time they begin to grow a
shell around this pitiful store of knowledge and wisdom, and
from then on they resist with enormous energy any attempts to
pierce that shell with anything new. In a world that is changing
so rapidly that even the most agile-minded cannot keep up with
all its ramifications, the effect of this shell-building is to develop
in a person a dislike—even perhaps a hatred—of the unfamiliar,
simply because it was not present in time to be included within
the shell. This hardening of the mind—psychosclerosis—is a long
distance from a child's acceptance and flexibility and openmindedness.

In recent years in Western industrialized countries, and to some
extent even in the not-so-affluent other parts of the world, the
cult of youth has taken over a large segment of society. It has
come to be a kind of secular religion, and it has certainly given
rise to—and in a circular way is also a result of—a multibillion-
dollar industry. Youth is considered—by the young, at least, and
a substantial number of their elders—the ideal time of life; to be
young is believed to be the most desirable age of all.

It was not always true. Through the Victorian period and lasting until some time after World War II, in Britain and Western
Europe as well as in the United States, to be old was to be

revered. Governments were run by graybeards, the armies and navies were commanded by elderly generals and admirals, and rulers of empires—Emperor Franz-Joseph and Queen Victoria—were venerated not so much for their nearness to God as for their age and longevity. The world's business was conducted by old men, and families were subject to the wills of their oldest members.

Young and middle-aged men in that period were considered too youthful, too inexperienced, too lacking in wisdom, too foolish even, to take primary responsibility for important matters. And these men consulted their fathers or other older men on all significant decisions even in their personal lives, and would no more have failed to defer to these men than they would have failed to stand to attention when the National Anthem was being played.

Women, of course, suffered under this regime even more than men, because daughters were considered even more immature, more vulnerable, and more dependent than sons, and therefore in greater need of supervision and protection throughout their lives. Women who thought for themselves were rare during that period, and women who acted for themselves, without the consent of parents, guardians, husbands, or other "wiser" heads, were rarer still.

The raising of children in such an atmosphere was certain to be damaging to the children. Childhood was seen as a difficult period that was unfortunately necessary for the production of mature, no-nonsense adults, and the entire effort of the education and training of children was aimed at making adults of them as soon as possible. Thus the "ladylike" little girl and the "gentlemanly" little boy. The closer their behavior to that of adults, the better. As a practical matter this meant that children were expected to demonstrate quiet good manners; respect for anyone older (thus wiser) than themselves; conscientiousness in all duties, of which there were many; willingness to study even the most uninteresting material because it was "good for them"; and an unquestioned obedience to all rules of the adult world. "It doesn't matter what you teach a boy, so long as he doesn't want to learn it," said one leading educator of the period.

Imagination was frowned upon—feared, even—curiosity was

derided ("Curiosity killed the cat!"), free playfulness and humor were discouraged, openmindedness was thought to be heretical, and honesty was often considered simple rudeness. As for the most precious of all childlike qualities, the eagerness to learn, it was accepted by adults only so long as the subject of the learning was a "proper" one; otherwise it was forbidden.

Children who failed to thrive under this Spartan regime were themselves blamed for their failure. It occurred only to a few people that perhaps the fault lay in the failure of the adult world to understand the nature of childhood, and in fact in the failure to understand the development of human beings.

We have made some progress in this understanding over the past fifty years. Anthropologists, psychologists, other social scientists, and even some educators have begun to recognize that children are not simply small imperfect adults who must be dragged as early as possible into the adult-behaving world. We know that children are developing human beings who will continue developing all their lives if they are not prevented. And now we begin to see that the goal of life is to die young—as late as possible.

The principle of neoteny has much to teach us about the behavior of human beings, children and adults. Its history is a long one, much too long to include in its entirety here, but a brief account will help us to understand its nature and its ramifications. A more complete discussion is included in Appendix A.

The early work on neoteny was entirely concerned with the physical evolution and development of organisms, and with the discovery that certain physical traits that are characteristic of the fetus or of an immature stage of life of some specific creature are sometimes retained into the adult stage. The word was coined in 1884 by Julius Kollmann, Professor of Zoology at the University of Basel, in order to describe the process of transformation whereby newts and similar creatures mature sexually while they are still in larval form.

One would hardly expect that this discovery, which had been made some twenty years before Kollman named it, would lead directly to a belief that human beings are designed to retain into adulthood many of the behavioral traits that characterize human childhood. And, indeed, it was some years before the concept of neoteny was applied to human beings at all, and then only to their physical endowment. Havelock Ellis, that great liberator of the human spirit, without knowing of Kollmann's work or the work of his predecessors, was the first person to apply the idea of neoteny to human beings when, in 1894, he pointed out that the fetuses and young of apes and of human beings are much more alike than are the adults of the two groups. Furthermore, both are much more like adult human beings than they are like adult apes.

Louis Bolk, Professor of Anatomy at the University of Amsterdam, put a name to this tendency. In 1926 he pointed out that compared with other primates, the rate of development of humans, from fetus through infancy and childhood into adulthood, is slow, and that adult humans exhibit many physical traits that are also features of the human fetus. This is not so true of the adults of other animals. He listed flat-facedness, minimum body hair, large brain size, structure of hands and feet, the form of the pelvis, and a number of additional physical characteristics that change in other animals but that in human beings persist into adulthood. In short, said Bolk, echoing Kollmann, "Man, in his bodily development, is a primate fetus that has become sexually mature." Bolk called this principle "fetalization." Fetalization was effected by retardation of the rate of development.

The importance of this slow development, or retardation, was seen by J. B. S. Haldane, as it was by Bolk, as a major evolutionary trend in human beings. In 1932 he underscored the fact that the essential feature of the latest stage of human evolution has been not the acquisition of new features but rather the preservation of embryonic and infantile traits that had been developed when the organisms were in the womb sheltered from violence. The retention of these features has enabled human beings, Haldane suggested, to shed much of their animalism; Haldane further proposed that if human evolution is to continue along the same lines, "it will probably involve a still greater prolongation of childhood and retardation of maturity."

Konrad Lorenz, German ethologist, writing in 1950, maintained that by far the more important features in the history of human evolution are not physical but behavioral. He drew heav-

ily on the ideas of German sociologist Arnold Gehlen, who recognized as early as 1940 that the unique and outstanding human
trait is that of remaining in an unending state of development.
The specialty of humans is nonspecialization, versatility; they
have remained free to change as change is required by whatever
environment they encounter; they are able to develop special
traits to meet special needs. Lorenz holds that these traits are
behavioral as well as physical.

Physical and behavioral qualities are inextricably intertwined.
The size of the brain, the agility of the limbs, posture, the structure of hands and feet, the position of eyes and ears all make
possible, or impossible, certain ways of behaving. And these
features have been determined for each creature by the evolutionary process that has produced it and its kind. Therefore,
before we discuss specific behavior patterns it is necessary to
understand the development of physical patterns, through the
evolution of the species. Only then can we understand something
of the manner in which behavior potentialities evolved, even
though physical and behavioral development have evolved under
totally different selection pressures.

Terminology

It has been said that definitions are not really meaningful at the
beginning of an inquiry, that they can only be so at the end of
one, but at this juncture I think we are ready for some simple
definitions. Viola, in *Twelfth Night,* remarks, "Nay, that's cer-
taine: they that dally nicely with words, may quickly make them
wanton." It is characteristic of early stages in the development
of a scientific idea that those who come upon it independently
usually invent their own terms by which to describe it. The result
frequently is that such terms take on lives of their own and what
was once a single specific idea assumes many different forms.
This often leads to years of muddled thinking and tiresome confusion. I shall not take the reader's time by entering into a discussion of this phenomenon in connection with the idea of
neoteny. Professor Stephen Jay Gould has already ably done this
in his book *Ontogeny and Phylogeny* (1977), which has contrib-

uted greatly to the introduction of order into a backwater of science that might well have been described as awash in the systematics of confusion.

Since Professor Gould and I are for the most part in agreement on these matters and on the important role neoteny has played in the evolution of humans, it may be helpful if at this point the terms that have thus far been used shall be clearly defined.

Paedomorphosis is the process whereby the fetal and/or juvenile traits of ancestors or own-species or subspecies ("races") are retained into later stages of individual development.

Neoteny has precisely the same meaning as paedomorphosis. The definitions usually given of both processes represent a distinction without a difference, and since this is so the two terms will be used interchangeably.

The only respect in which these definitions differ from earlier ones is that to the traits of ancestors appearing in later stages of development in paedomorphism Gould and I have added also those of fetal and juvenile members of the species, so the terms also refer to traits that appear in adult humans that are characteristic of their own fetal or juvenile forms. For example, as many independent investigators have observed, the juvenile skulls of such prehistoric hominids as the African humanlike form *Australopithecus africanus,* the pithecanthropine *Homo erectus* (formerly known as *Pithecanthropus erectus*), and Neandertal man exhibit many features that more closely resemble those of modern man than they do those of their own adult forms. (See Figure 14.) Modern humans could have evolved from neandertaloids by the simple retention of the juvenile traits of these forms; that is to say, by neoteny.

In this manner the neotenous forms would come to look more like grown-up juveniles than the more specialized forms from which they had evolved. The specialized forms when young were once juvenile-looking too, but as they grew older they developed heavy browridges, large teeth, projecting jaws, and the like. This process is the opposite of paedomorphism, and is known as *gerontomorphism* (Gr. *geron* = old man, and *morphosis* = development of form, becoming like an old individual, meaning extreme specialization). Gerontomorphosis is a form of

evolution by specialization of the adult stages of successive independent developments. Its net effect is to decrease ability for
further evolution and to expose species to extinction.

The adults of the great apes—orangutan, chimpanzee, and
gorilla—are all gerontomorphic forms (Figure 1), as are most prehistoric humans up to the Upper Pleistocene, some thirty thousand years ago. Humans are born at an earlier stage of physical
development than apes, and as they develop remain more like
the immature infant than does the ape, the latter pursuing a more
specialized developmental path. The human infant starts off by
being born with a heavier body than the ape, and a head size that
in proportion to body size is relatively the same as in the ape; but
in proportion to their height the apes end up with a heavier body
and proportionately smaller head. In other words, the apes di-
verge from what would seem to be the promise of their infant
traits and develop instead toward gerontomorphy, whereas humans retain that early promise and continue to develop by
stretching out their juvenility for many years. This is brought out
in Figure 2, which makes graphically clear the neoteny of the
skull. The figure shows the growth of the chimpanzee skull (*left*)
compared with the human skull plotted on transformed coordinates, showing the relative displacement of parts. At the fetal
stage (*top*), the chimpanzee and human skulls are much more
alike than they are at the adult stage (*bottom*). It will be seen that
the adult human skull departs far less from its fetal form than
does the chimpanzee skull at the same stage of development.
Indeed, when one superimposes a drawing of the human adult
skull over one of a newborn human's, it is seen that the adult
human skull for the most part simply represents an enlarged
newborn's and is little altered in proportions (Figure 3). When
one compares the growth of the newborn ape skull (in this case
the orangutan) with that of the human (Figure 4), it can readily
be seen that there is a tremendous forward growth of the ape face
and jaws and very little growth of the brainbox compared with
the human. In the gorilla this kind of gerontomorphic development in the adult skull compared with its juvenile form is even
more striking. The marked extent to which the adult chimpanzee
departs from the promise of its juvenile form is equally notable,
if not more so, when the living juvenile chimpanzee is compared
with its adult form (Figure 5). From these striking photographs it

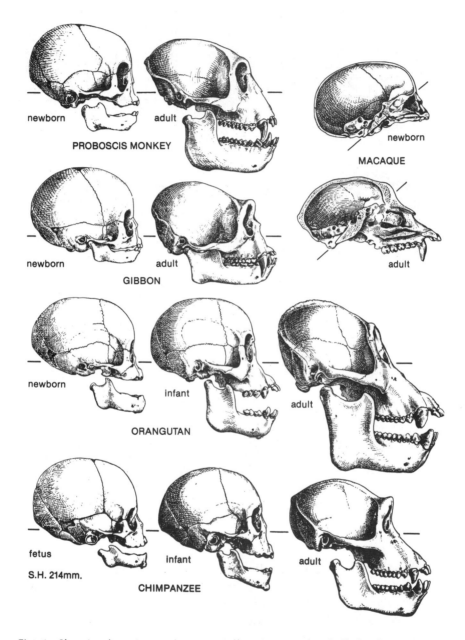

newborn   adult

PROBOSCIS MONKEY

newborn

MACAQUE

adult

newborn   adult

GIBBON

newborn   infant   adult

ORANGUTAN

fetus

S.H. 214mm.   infant   adult

CHIMPANZEE

Fig. 1. Showing how in monkeys as well as in apes the skull develops into a gerontomorphic form in the adult. (After Schultz)

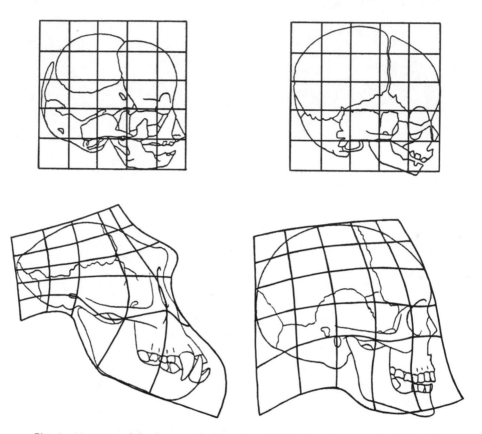

Fig. 2. Neoteny of the human skull made evident when the growth of the chimpanzee skull (*left*) and of the human skull (*right*) are plotted on transformed coordinates, which show the relative displacement of each part. The chimpanzee and the human skulls are much more alike at the fetal stage (*top*) than they are at the adult stage (*bottom*). The adult human skull also departs less from the fetal form than the adult chimpanzee skull departs from its fetal form, except in the case of the chin, which becomes relatively larger in human beings. The growth of the chin is due to the differential rate of growth of different parts of the jaw—the tooth-bearing part being slowed down while the chin portion continues to grow. (After Lewontin)

will be evident how closely the juvenile chimpanzee resembles both the human child *and* adult human. From such a juvenile chimpanzee it would require very few changes by neoteny to produce a human form. Indeed, the chimpanzee, and especially a form resembling the pygmy chimpanzee of Zaire, in equatorial Africa, seems increasingly likely as a possible ancestor of the

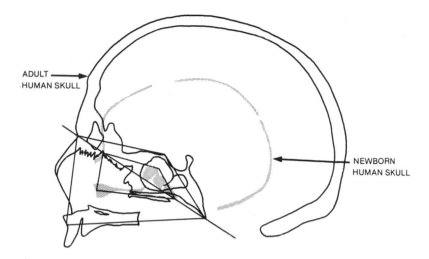

Fig. 3. Midsection outlines of the newborn human and adult human skulls, showing, except for increase in size of the adult skull, there is no significant change in form from newborn to adult.

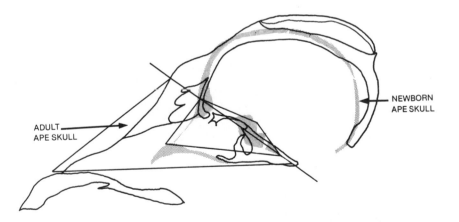

Fig. 4. Showing the great change in form from newborn to adult in the ape, in this case the orangutan.

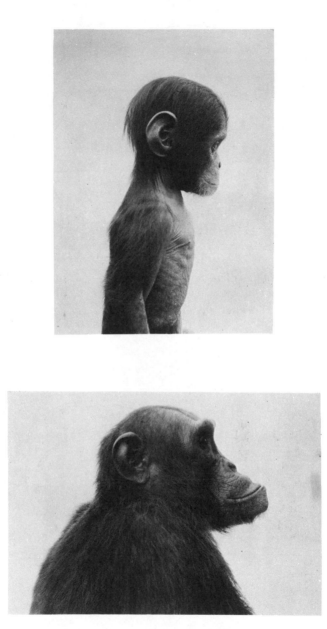

Fig. 5. Showing how humanlike the juvenile chimpanzee is compared with its adult form.

earliest humanlike forms. Dr. Adrienne Zihlman and her colleagues at the Department of Anthropology at the University of California in Santa Cruz, who have carefully studied the rare skeletal remains of the pygmy chimpanzee (*Pan paniscus*) as well as the characteristics of living members of the species, find that they move as easily on the ground as they do in the trees. In captivity they seem to walk upright more often than the common chimpanzee. In addition they are more generalized than other apes in their morphological traits, not having developed long arms for hanging and swinging. Their canine teeth, brain size, and body size show fewer differences between the sexes than is the case in the other apes. In these respects the pygmy chimps more closely approach humans than they do other apes.

In their chromosomal structure, humans and chimpanzees are remarkably alike. The genetic changes accounting for the morphological differences between humans and chimpanzees may be quite small. A few regulatory genes, through enzymatic processes, may have large somatic effects, whereas the remaining structural genes may be time-dependent in their rate of fixation, and of little selective significance. Hence, neoteny would not have much work to do in order to transform an ape into a human. Nevertheless, in spite of their genetic resemblance to humans, chimpanzees remain closer in form and behavior to apes than to humans.

In paedomorphosis there is a displacement of ancestral features to later stages of development. Certain ancestral traits are, as it were, "pushed off" the end of individual development. As Julian Huxley put it, "Previous adult characters . . . never appear because their formation is too long delayed: they are lost to the species by being driven off the time-scale of its development." And, again, in another work, "The old adult characters may be swept off the map and be replaced by characters of a quite novel type." It is not that one trait is displaced from one locus to another, but that it is either wholly or partially discarded or substantively modified. We have already mentioned as an example the replacement of the greatly developed brow ridges of early humans by the smooth supraorbital region of the fetus and child. The body hair of our anthropoid ancestors has only been partially replaced by a relatively hairless skin, whereas the lower extremities have gone on growing at an accelerated rate.

1

Neoteny and the Biological Evolution of Humankind

> It is the possibility of escaping from the blind alleys of specialization into a new period of plasticity and adaptive radiation which makes the idea of paedomorphosis so attractive in evolutionary theory. Both its possibilities and limitations deserve the most careful exploration.
>
> —JULIAN HUXLEY
> *The Evolutionary Process* 1954

> The unique human trait of always remaining in a state of development is quite certainly a gift that we owe to the neotenous nature of mankind.
>
> —KONRAD LORENZ
> *Part and Parcel in Animal and Human Societies*

In surveying the development of the concept of neoteny it becomes clear that the morphological changes in the varieties of humankind have been mainly brought about by the retention into adult life of traits principally characteristic of the fetus. As Sir Arthur Keith, the distinguished English anatomist and anthropologist, put it, the outstanding structural peculiarities of humankind have been produced during the embryonic and fetal stages of its evolutionary history. It is not so much embryonic as fetal traits, however, that are neotenized both in the evolutionary and individual development of humans. In the evolution of humankind from an anthropoid stock it is easy to see that gradual change from anthropoid to human could have come about by the retention of the generalized fetal form of the anthropoid into adult age.

Such retention of anthropoid fetal traits would come about in a mosaic manner—that is to say, not all fetal ancestral traits would be retained in descendent forms, but only one or a few at a time. For example, in the australopithecines the front teeth (incisors and canines) underwent reduction, while the teeth at the sides and back of the jaws (premolars and molars) retained their large size, undergoing reduction only at a later time. The premaxillary diastema, the space between the canine (eyetooth) and the first premolar for the reception of the projecting canine of the lower jaw, remained quite wide in the juvenile australopithecine (Figure 6), and was reduced in later australopithecines. In the pithecanthropines (*Homo erectus*), a group that may well have originated from the australopithecine stock, the premaxillary

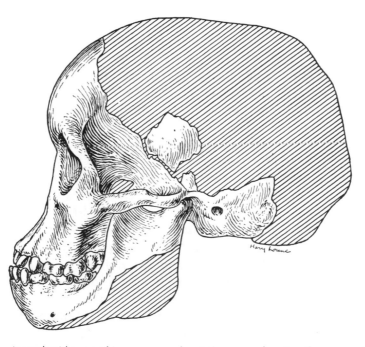

Fig. 6. *Australopithecus africanus,* age about six years, showing the premaxillary diastema in the upper jaw.

diastema is present in the earliest of them, *Homo erectus robust-us,* even though it is clear that the canine of the lower jaw had undergone reduction. In short, the space in the upper jaw remained, though it no longer served any useful purpose. In later members of the pithecanthropines the diastema completely disappeared. Another example of mosaic evolution (see pp. 257 and 270) is that while erect posture was attained by the australopithecines, brain size in the early forms did not appear to change much from that of their anthropoid ancestors. From *Homo erectus* to Neandertal man, through Solo man of Java, to modern man (*Homo sapiens sapiens*), we proceed by a steplike process to shed one anthropoid trait after another: the large teeth, projecting jaws, cranial crests, massive eyebrow-ridges and facial structures. Simply by stretching out the fetal stages of development, and accelerating the rate of development of the brain, the trend is toward the retention of the structural traits of an ancestral fetus. The course followed in the structural evolution of humankind is schematically shown in Figures 7 and 8. In Figure 7 in the first column we see the skulls of newborn primates ranging from the rhesus monkey (*Macaca mulatta*) to a European human. We see that all of them closely resemble one another. But reading from the bottom row across from the newborn to the adult male in the last column, one can see that in the case of monkey and ape there is a marked change from paedomorphic to gerontomorphic form. Evidence of gerontomorphism becomes progressively much less marked in the human forms, Neandertal, Australian aborigine, and European. Indeed, in these latter forms as one progresses from Neandertal to European the trend is markedly toward paedomorphism, the maintenance of the juvenile form of the skull. This would be even more strikingly evident were it possible to show a series of Chinese skulls ranging from newborn to adult males, for in the adult Chinese skull paedomorphism has proceeded further than in any other people. The Mongoloid skull generally, whether Chinese or Japanese, has been rather more neotenized than the Caucasoid or European (Table I). The female skull, it will be noted, is more paedomorphic in all human populations than the male skull; this also holds true for many other somatic traits, and, I have not the least doubt, for functional and behavioral

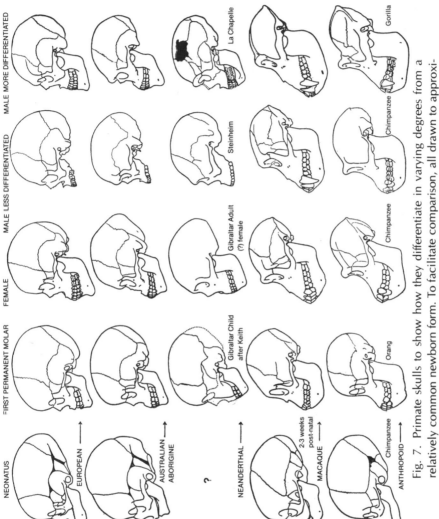

Fig. 7. Primate skulls to show how they differentiate in varying degrees from a relatively common newborn form. To facilitate comparison, all drawn to approximately the same size. (After Abbie)

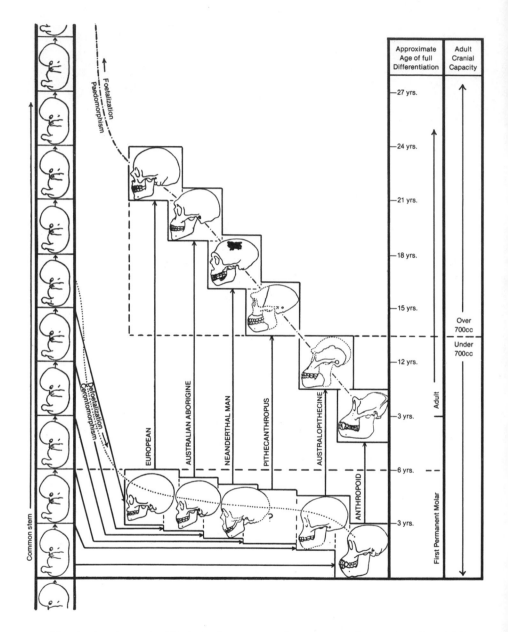

Fig. 8. A scheme to illustrate the suggested common primate stem in which distinctive forms of various primates have been derived from it by a combination of the processes of gerontomorphism and paedomorphism. (After Abbie)

TABLE I

Neotenous Structural Traits in Which Mongoloids and Negroids Differ from Caucasoids

Mongoloids	*Negroids*	*Bushman-Hottentot*
Larger brain	Flattish nose	Light skin pigment
Larger braincase	Flat root of the	Less hairy
Broader skull	nose	Large brain
Broader face	Small ears	Round-headed
Flat root of the nose	Narrower joints	Bulging forehead
Inner eye fold	Frontal skull	Small cranial
More protuberant eyes	eminences	sinuses
Lack of brow ridges	Later closure of pre-	Flat root of nose
Greater delicacy of bones	maxillary	Small face
Shallow mandibular fossa	sutures	Small mastoid
Small mastoid processes	Less hairy	processes
Stocky build	Longer eyelashes	Wide eye separa-
Persistence of thymus	Cruciform pattern	tion
gland into adult life	of lower sec-	Median eye fold
Persistence of juvenile	ond and third	Short stature
form of zygomatic	molars	Horizontal penis
muscle		
Persistence of juvenile		
form of superior lip		
muscle		
Later eruption of full den-		
tition (except second		
and third molars)		
Less hairy		
Fewer sweat glands		
Fewer hairs per		
square centimeter		
Long torso		

traits as well (see Table II). In other words, the female realizes the promise of the species rather more fully than the male.

In Table III I have listed some thirty neotenous physical traits in humans; some of these are obviously a reflection of others. For example, the globular form of the skull reflects the great

---

TABLE II
Neotenous Traits of Female as Compared with Those of Male

More delicately constructed skeleton
All protuberances, tuberosities, and ridges, such as external occipital
    protuberance, roughnesses for the attachment of ligaments,
    mastoid processes, eyebrow ridges, and the like, greatly
    reduced
Narrower joints
Larger brain in relation to total body size
Less hairy
More delicate skin
Smaller body size
Greater longevity
Basal metabolism 5 to 7 percent lower in female
Heartbeat faster by some seven beats per minute
Greater extension of developmental periods
Larger size of tears
Voice more highly pitched

---

increase in the size of the brain, while flatness of face, small
jaws, and small teeth are closely related to one another.

Neotenous functional or physiological traits in humans are
many. Except for behavioral traits, these are listed in Table IV.

The Cranial Flexure

In the embryo of all mammals and most vertebrates, Bolk
pointed out, the axis of the head forms a right angle with that of
the trunk; this is known as the *cranial flexure*. In all mammals,
with the exception of humans, a rotation of the head occurs
during the later stages of development so that the head assumes
an orientation that is continuous with the direction of the
backbone, as for example in the adult dog (Figure 9). Humans,
on the other hand, retain the cranial flexure, the face pointing in
the direction of the body. The visual axis, the line of sight, of
both dog and human is horizontal; however, the dog's body is

also horizontal while that of humans is vertical. In the adult great apes the position of the body is in between, being obliquely quadrupedal, and the axis of the head is also intermediate; the foramen magnum, the hole at the base of the skull through which the spinal cord passes down into the vertebral canal, is situated rather more posteriorly than the central position it occupies in either fetal ape or human. It thus transpires that the human erect posture represents the retention in postnatal development of a fetal condition, that is, a horizontal visual axis and a vertical or perpendicular body.

Against the view that human erect bipedalism has been made possible by the retention of a neotenous fetal relationship between the cranial flexure and body axis, it has been argued that changes in the pelvic girdle, the lower extremity, and foot, and the differences in muscular attachments, especially the gluteus

---

TABLE III
Neotenous Physical Traits in Humans

Cranial flexure	Large braincase
Head situated over top of spine	Small teeth
Forward position of foramen magnum	Late eruption of teeth
	Prominent nose
Forward position of occipital condyles	Absence of cranial crests
	Thinness of skull bones
Lack of heavy brow ridges	Gracile skeleton
Orbits under cranial cavity	Thin nails
Flatness of face (orthognathy)	Nonrotation of big toe
Contact between sphenoid and ethmoid bones in anterior cranial cavity	Relative hairlessness of body
	Lack of pigment in some groups
	Curvature of pelvic axis
Retarded closure of cranial sutures	Lack of pronounced physical differences
Large size of brain	Anterior position of vagina
Round-headedness (fetal head index 72–82)	Downward direction of vagina
	Persistence of labia majora
Small jaws	Persistence of hymen
Small face	Persistence of penile prepuce

TABLE IV
Neotenous Functional Traits in Humans

Rapid growth of brain well into third year
Low birth weight
External gestation
Prolonged immaturity
Prolonged dependency
Infant's great need of fluids (150 ml per day)
Fetal rate of body growth, weight, and length during first year
Prolonged growth period
Ends of long and phalangeal bones remain cartilaginous for years
Lack of estrus period (sexual periodicity)
Late descent of testes
Late development of secondary sexual traits
Late development of spermatogenesis
Late development of menstruation
Late development of ovulation
Late development of reproductive maturity

maximus (the large muscle of the buttock), render it unlikely that neoteny in this connection has any explanatory value whatever. In the first place, it is said, such modifications are never present in the apes, in either embryos or fetuses, or at any other stage of development; and in the second place, some of these traits are not even to be found in fetal humans. Furthermore, a fundamental feature of the erect bipedal human is the elongated lower extremity, a trait the very opposite of neotenous.

All these criticisms of Bolk's views are quite sound, but they do not in the least weaken his main argument, for he did not claim that erect bipedalism came into being as a sudden mutation. On the contrary, he appears to have understood that the development of the erect posture was quite gradual. However that may be, the hypothesis of neoteny does not exclude the operation of other factors in the development of the erect bipedal form of locomotion.

When we look at our contemporary primate relatives, the orangutan, chimpanzee, and gorilla, and observe the various

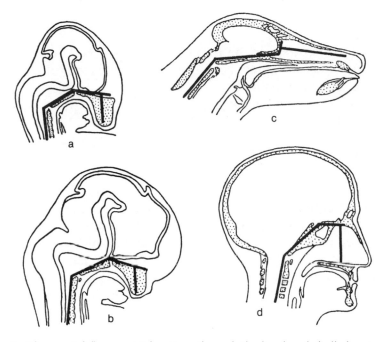

Fig. 9. The cranial flexure. Midsections through the head and skull showing the angle the head makes with the trunk in **a** embryo dog; **b** embryo human; **c** adult dog; and **d** adult human. (After Bolk, 1926)

postures they assume under different conditions, including erect ones, we experience no difficulty in reconstructing the stages through which our ancestors must have progressed to achieve our own erect bipedal posture.

Bolk also drew attention to the fact that the cranial flexure in adult humans is paralleled by what de Beer termed the pubic flexure. In the embryo of mammals the axis of the urogenital structures and rectum is directed downward; but in the adult mammal, with the exception of humans, the axis of these structures undergoes rotation so that it comes to lie parallel with the backbone, resulting in a backward direction of the vaginal aperture. By contrast, in humans the fetal orientation of these structures is retained, so that the vaginal aperture is directed downward, a principal effect of which is the standard horizontal face-to-face posture in copulation.

The Position of the Foramen Magnum

The central position of the foramen magnum (the large aperture through which the spinal cord passes) at the base of the skull is another unique human feature among the primates. Interestingly, in infant nonhuman primates this foramen is more centrally situated than it is in adults. In these animals, during the growth of the skull—especially of the jaws and face—and the eruption of the teeth, the structure that contributes to the posterior and lateral margins of the foramen, the occipital bone, is pushed, as it were, backward and upward, so that the axis of the foramen frequently ends up facing backward almost in the vertical plane. One of our early progenitors in the line from the pithecanthropines to Neandertal man, and so on to ourselves—namely, Solo man from Java—possessed a foramen magnum not quite as centrally situated as in modern humans, the anterior part of which was in the horizontal plane, while the posterior half was almost in the vertical plane. In suckling apes and humans the central portion of the foramen magnum is probably associated with the need for the head to be positioned erectly in nursing at the mother's breast. Here, too, a flat face is an advantage, owing to the peculiar mechanics of the breastfeeding situation. It is for the same reason that the jaws remain undeveloped in all suckling nonhuman primate infants who, like the baboons, will later develop considerable muzzles. Toward the end of the suckling period in the monkeys and apes, when weaning is usually commenced, the changes in the face and base of the skull lead to the gradual positioning and orientation of the foramen posteriorly. In humans the fetal position and orientation of the foramen remain unchanged. Hence, the infantile stage of development of these traits, as Sir Arthur Keith pointed out, has become permanent in humans.

It might be thought, judging from the conditions prevailing in contemporary gatherer-hunter peoples, that the prolonged and intensive breastfeeding enjoyed by children in prehistoric societies, generally lasting some four to seven or more years, had some relation to the development of the erect posture in humans. However, since under natural conditions chimpanzees breastfeed for some five years, the principal factors operative in producing the erect posture have to be looked for elsewhere.

The Face and the Flexure

The bones of the face develop quite independently of those of the rest of the skull. The facial bones are the nasal, maxillary (upper jaw), zygomatic (cheekbones), and mandible (lower jaw) (Figure 10). The other large cranial bones contribute to the formation of the brainbox and the sides, back, and base of the skull. The frontal bone also makes its contribution to the face as well as to the sides and base of the skull. The facial bones tend to be vertically inclined in humans, whereas in apes these bones tend to project in a more obliquely forward direction, largely as a result of the projection of the jaws, a condition called *progna-*

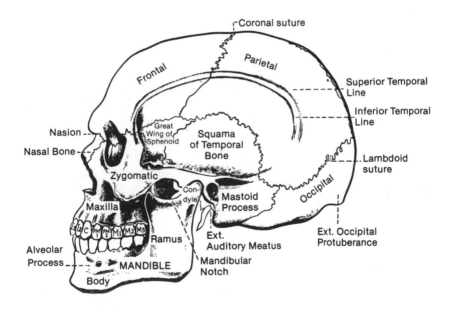

Fig. 10. Human adult skull.

thism. In the development of early fetal primates, conditions are quite different; with their cranial flexure, the anterior portion of the base of the skull is inclined downward, and the face is similarly inclined beneath the base. In the course of fetal development, however, the flexure straightens out, resulting in the apparent projecting jaws characteristic of all primates with the exception of humans. In humans the fetal flexure is retained, and it is this neotenous condition that accounts for the orthognathy or flat-facedness of humans. These views, using somewhat different terms, were set out by Bolk in a paper entitled "The Problem of Orthognathism" in 1923.

Since orthognathy is confined to the early fetal stages of development in the apes, the neotenous mutations that led to orthognathy must have occurred fairly early in hominid evolution.

The Nose

There is one feature of the human face that seems rather puzzling. It is the nose. The human nose is unique among primates, for it juts out from the face alone like a peninsula left behind by the retreating, verticalizing face. It would seem that in the rush to reduce the prognathic jaws, there was a failure to deal with the excess material that remained after the rearrangement of the facial bones. But that is not exactly what happened. Since prognathism makes possible a considerable surface area of vitally necessary mucous membrane within the nasal fossa and its associated structures, reduction of the jaws together with the mucous membranes of the nasal fossa would have constituted a selectively great disadvantage. Hence, the mucous membrane was retained by projecting it outward under cover of that complex organ we call the nose. Whether flat, long, broad, or narrow, whatever its shape, as long as the surface area of the mucous membrane remains adequate for the important functions it is called upon to perform during every moment of the individual's life, it matters not one bit what the external form of the nose may be.

If the nose does not appear to be a neotenous trait, *that* is appearance only, for it has developed by retardation of the growth of the jaws and a retraction and rotation outward of the frontal processes of the upper jaw. This rotation comes about as if by crowding, so that the paired nasal bones, which are attached laterally to the frontal processes of the maxillary bones ascending upward from the jawbones, are also pushed outward, thus producing for the first time in the primates the elevated form of the nasal bones; these, together with the median septal cartilage, result in the human nose. So the human nose, if not itself a neotenous trait in the sense of having been retained by retardation from an earlier stage, is certainly the consequence of such a process affecting neighboring structures.

Dr. E. V. Glanville, in a study of nose shape, prognathism, and adaptation, found that with increasing prognathism there was an increase in the broadness of the nose. With retardation of jaw growth the jaws, as it were, withdrew, leaving the nasal aperture and the nose itself narrower and more prominent. Hence, we may conclude that the nose constitutes yet another example of the workings of neoteny.

The Sense of Smell

It has often been stated that humans have a poor sense of smell. This is quite untrue. The human infant is born with an acute sense of smell, and when only a few days old is quickly able to distinguish the odor of his own mother's breastpad (the pad worn next to the mother's breast in the brassiere) from that taken from any other breastfeeding mother. Olfactory ability is far from contemptible in humans, and in a number of respects is not far below that of the dog. Compared, however, with that of the dog, the olfactory epithelium is much reduced in humans; nevertheless olfactory efficiency remains quite considerable into adult life, and thus the ability to smell as well as we do may be regarded as a non-neotenous function of a neotenous nasal structure. Far from becoming vestigial, as is sometimes claimed, the sense of smell plays an important adaptive role in alerting humans to the presence of a large variety of otherwise undetectable conditions.

It is conceivable that the nose would have remained exactly as

it is in the apes had its projection not served some adaptively
more useful purpose than olfaction. Had the nose not developed
its prominence with the retraction of the jaws, it would have
suffered a significant loss of the mucous membrane that lines the
nasal and associated cavities. This would have resulted in a serious loss of the many advantages afforded by a large number of
physiological functions performed by the nasal mucous membrane. With the prominent nose and its median nasal septum
dividing the nasal cavity into two parts, the surface area covered
by the mucosa is greatly enlarged.

The nasal mucous membrane is richly endowed with secretory
cells which not only serve to supply the continuously moving
blanket which nourishes the cilia that move it, but also carry
along with it such substances as lysozyme, which are lethal to
viruses and bacteria. In this manner the integrity of the mucous
membrane is preserved and harmful viruses and bacteria disposed of. The rich vascular net of the nasal mucosa together with
the secretions of the mucosal cells, a secretion of almost one
quart a day, helps to maintain the relative humidity of the in-
haled air at 95 percent, and its temperature at body level. Add to
all these arrangements the hairs guarding the entrance to the
nasal cavities and our view of the size and functions of the nose
begins to make some adaptive sense.

Weeping

Among the infrahuman primates the infant is carried about clinging to its mother's fur, mother and infant are in close contact,
and mother is always within reach. In humans there is no comforting soft fur to cling to, and during the day the infant may
often be separated from the mother or other caretaker. Under
such circumstances whenever the infant experiences a need that
is not immediately satisfied he will cry out loudly for attention,
until his mother or someone else satisfies his need. The infant
ape clinging to its mother's fur, needs only to seek out the breast
to have most of its needs satisfied.

The human infant who is not in his mother's arms may have no
other means of drawing attention to his needs than crying. Were
the infant's needs adequately satisfied it is highly probable he

would not cry at all. There is no sound so compelling as the cry of the dependent infant, and there is little doubt that this development in the human infant was soon followed by another, namely, weeping.

It is a curious fact that humans are the only creatures who weep—weeping being defined as the shedding of tears during emotional distress or joy. Weeping has been attributed to other animals, but the truth is that psychic weeping is not known to occur as a normal function in any other creature. Students of the primates have uniformly failed to observe anything resembling weeping in any nonhuman primate. The great student of primate behavior Robert Yerkes wrote, "Young anthropoid apes frequently cry under certain circumstances which would induce like response in the human infant and child, but never in such instances even when the response is extreme have I seen tears."

The age at which human infants begin to cry with tears varies considerably. Some infants are able to do so at or shortly after birth, while others fail to do so until they are eight weeks of age. The average age at which tears begin to accompany emotional distress is between five and six weeks. The peak of the ability to weep is reached in childhood, between six and nine years, and gradually tapers off in adulthood. The late development of weeping in the human infant would suggest that it is a trait that developed some time after the assumption of human status. What factor or combination of factors, then, was it in the evolution of early humans that may have been responsible for the appearance of weeping?

The length of the dependency period of the human child at once suggests itself. During the earlier part of that dependency period the human infant is without speech or the ability to help himself.

> An infant crying in the night:
> An infant crying for the light:
> And with no language but a cry.

The infant's principal means of attracting attention to his needs when in distress is by crying. Crying is essentially an activity involving the respiratory system and glottis, the muscle systems subserving these, the facial muscles, changes in arterial blood pressure, central nervous system changes, changes in metabolism, and the loss of heat. Babies cry with their eyelids firmly closed. The harder they cry the firmer the closure of the eyelids. The function of this is to oppose the pressure of the conjunctival and deeper vessels of the eye. If the pressure of the eyelids for some reason is prevented or relaxed, breakages in the small vessels could occur, as sometimes happens in sudden explosive coughs, sneezing, and even in yawning and laughter.

Prolonged crying can be dangerous if it is not accompanied by tears. Even a short spell of tearless crying in a young infant is likely to have a desiccating effect on the mucous membranes of the nose and throat. This can easily be shown by comparing the appearance of these mucous membranes in infants crying tearlessly with those of infants who cry with tears. The mucous membranes of the former appear to be excessively dry; ciliary action appears to have ceased; and there is a considerable congestion of mucous membrane blood vessels with obvious breakages in many.

Excessive intake and expulsion of air even in adults will quickly dry mucous membranes, and it is this intake and expulsion of air in the tearless crying infant that I see as closely associated with the origin and development of weeping. The mucous membrane begins at the entrance of the nose and lines the structures of the nasal cavity and throat.

It is the mucous membrane of the nose that constitutes the most immediate contact of the respiratory system with the external world. No other living cells are directly exposed to the insults and assaults of the environment. The nasal mucous membrane must withstand the impact of respired air laden with viruses, bacteria, dust, other particles, and gases. Discharges from the eye enter by the nasolacrimal ducts, which lead from the median corners of the eyes, and trickle back over the mucous membrane. The air may be dry or moist, it may be at subzero temperature or very hot, and the respired air may vary rapidly from hot to cold. The mucous membrane is adapted to meet all these contingencies; however, dry air deprives the mucus of water and impairs its efficiency as a continuously moving protective blanket.

The bacteriocidal and bacteriostatic efficiency of the mucous membrane is considerable. It has been observed, for example, that 90 to 95 percent of viable bacteria placed on the nasal mucous membrane are inactivated in from five to ten minutes. The antiviral and antibacterial action of the mucous membrane is principally due to the action of lysozyme. When drying of the mucous membrane occurs the cilia tend to lose their function and soon die. This is followed by a piling up and drying of mucus, and the membrane becomes permeable. In this state the gelatinous mass of mucus becomes a hospitable culture medium for bacteria, which may then in large numbers pass through the nasal mucosa. The consequences of this process are not infrequently lethal.

I have proposed that in early humans weeping established itself as a trait of considerable adaptive value, serving to counteract the effects of tearless crying on the nasal mucosa of the infant. The dependent infants of early humans who cried for prolonged periods without benefit of tears would have stood much less chance of surviving than those who cried with tears. Crying with tears—weeping—serves to keep the mucous membrane wet and assists in maintaining as well as reinforcing its protective functions. It is an interesting fact that lysozyme, which is mainly responsible for the autosterilizing effect, is more concentrated in human tears than in the tears of any other higher mammal in which it is present. The tears of females are larger than those of males and contain more lysozyme, thus affording the female greater protection against bacteria and viruses.

From crying without to crying with tears there eventually develops the weeping of sympathy. Such sympathetic weeping is a social response. The universality of the capacity to weep in humans indicates the deep-seated biological basis of this behavioral trait. At the same time it indicates the existence of a profound biological basis for the feeling of sympathy that elicits weeping. Indeed, at every point, at every stage, and in every sector of human history, the outstanding characteristic humans have been called upon to exhibit has been sympathy, fellow-feeling, cooperation. In humans, especially, this combination of behavioral traits, prolonged as it is into all phases of later life, is neotenic. As Guthrie has pointed out, crying elicits protective behavior.

The crying adult becomes a child, and thereby tends to induce caring responses. Even callous males may find it difficult to resist a weeping female, and, until recently, most women, like many children, have known that a good cry may yield desired results. Emotional weeping in grief and sympathy constitutes a homeo-static mechanism designed to restore the organism to equilib-rium. We often weep tears of joy at some celebration or reunion with those we love. The Andaman Islanders make weeping an essential part of every social ceremony. When friends meet after a separation of a few weeks or longer, they greet each other by sitting down, one on the lap of the other, with arms around each other's necks, weeping and wailing for two or three minutes, till they are tired.

Between the tears of sorrow and those of joy there stretches a whole expanse of experiences in which humans weep. In almost every instance, whatever special state each may represent or communicate, the effect produced in the beholder is almost in-variably one of sympathy. A bond and an involvement are im-mediately established in a manner as instantaneous as it is pro-found, such as occurs with no other form of behavior.

It is suggested here that the sympathy evoked by weeping originated in the recognition by early humans of the meaning of weeping in the infant, and the identification of weeping as a signal of distress and an appeal for sympathy and succor; that, as humans evolved, the weeping and responses made to the child increasingly sensitized them to the emotional behavior of their fellow humans, the members of their community. Like the in-fant's cry, weeping at later stages is a signal for fellow feeling, for help, for aid and comfort. It is, therefore, for the most part something that is not, as a function, limited to the individual, but is a matter of the group, of the community, a form of behavior that is eminently evocative of response from others.

The emotional distress of which weeping is usually the exter-nal manifestation demands a delicacy of response of a peculiarly humane kind. It is, therefore, probable that weeping has exer-cised a humanizing effect upon humans as individuals, as per-sons, and also upon the human group as a community. In short, it seems likely that in the manner described, weeping—the flow of tears—has played a powerful role in the evolution of humans as compassionate creatures. Or to resume it all in the words of a great poet of nature, William Wordsworth, humankind is

> More skilful in self-knowledge, even more pure
> As tempted more; more able to endure,
> As more exposed to suffering and distress;
> Thence also more alive to tenderness.

The very fact that humans possess prominent noses suggests that they might do well to weep, or at least humidify them more often on those occasions when it would be appropriate to do so. In the English-speaking world a tabu has been imposed on weeping in boys. From an early age boys are informed that they are "little men" and must not cry—ever—for only girls and "sissies" do that. It is quite early made clear to "the little man" that if he cries he will lose the love of his parents and the respect of everyone else; hence, when he feels like crying, he represses the desire to do so, until in later life when he would wish to cry he often finds himself unable to do so. Meanwhile, his repressed weeping may be somatized, that is, expressed through the body, either in weeping through the skin in various eruptions, through the gastrointestinal tract in colitis or ulcers, through the respiratory tract in asthmatoid conditions, or in various other neurogenic symptoms. Weeping may be permitted in males on special occasions in the English-speaking world, as at wakes and funerals, but for the rest it is negatively sanctioned, interdicted. In such societies, weeping as a socially cohesive form of behavior has been lost.

Events are ordered otherwise among Romance-language–speaking peoples, and they appear to be the healthier for it. The display of emotion and weeping or tears among both sexes is expected on the occasions appropriate to them. What is considered a mark of weakness, and quite rightly an inhuman trait, is the *failure* to exhibit the expected emotional response—"the cold fish syndrome." In such cultures, in which weeping is considered normal, healthy behavior, there seems to be a great deal more human warmth, reflecting a more sensitive involvement in humanity generally.

Weeping contributes to the health of the individual, to his

humanity, and tends to deepen involvement in the welfare of
others.

What a waste of good nasal membrane it is, not to mention the
lacrimal and accessory lacrimal glands, that so many of the
long-nosed peoples of the world should fail to put them to use!

Forehead, Brow Ridges, Crests, Face, and Voice

The bulbous, prominent forehead is a trait characteristic of fetal
and infant apes and humans; but whereas this is soon lost in
apes, the prominent forehead is retained throughout life in humans. Moreover, as apes grow older they develop typical bony
prominences such as those over the orbits—the supraorbital
tori—as well as the sagittal and occipital crests on top of and at
the back of the skull, so markedly developed in the male gorilla
and the orang. There is a general development toward massive-
ness of the elements of the skull, especially of the upper and
lower jaws, and a general flattening of the frontal region immediately behind the supraorbital tori. In humans the tori never develop beyond ridges, and in most female skulls they do not develop at all. Such ridges are absent in the skulls of both sexes in
Mongoloid peoples. There are never any sagittal crests in humans (nor are there in chimpanzees), and the cranial bones are
less massive.

The general form of the forehead plays a highly significant role
in determining the appearance of the face, as well as the impression it makes upon us. We tend to associate a high forehead with
high intelligence, and a low one with low intelligence. We speak
of "highbrows" and "lowbrows." In fact, however, outside of
very general ranges, the form and shape of the forehead bear no
relation whatever to intelligence.

The various features most highly esteemed in that indefinable
esthetic judgment called feminine beauty in the early twentieth
century include a bulbous prominent forehead, a rather short,
retroussé nose set in a flat face between rounded cheeks, and
large eyes, presiding over full "cupid" lips—all fetal traits. The
"pin-up" girls and the typical Hollywood starlet and star con-
formed to this favored configuration. The predilection for this

kind of beauty was celebrated in an adenoidal popular song of the thirties entitled "Baby Face." Such females are the neotenized "babes" whom men often call by that name or by "baby." It is a term of endearment equivalent to the diminutives that occur in many languages, expressing smallness of size or lovableness or both. Konrad Lorenz most interestingly discussed the importance of rounded contours as a signal of childlikeness as compared with the rather more angular characteristics of adults. The neotenic features in the young combine to give the child its lovable or cuddly appearance, and to elicit in us a caring response (see Figure 11). Lorenz points out that the social effects of the neotenized appearance may, for example, be seen in the products of the doll industry—the result of much research and experiment—and also in the various types of animals, such as pug-dogs and Pekinese, that are sometimes adopted as pets by childless women as substitutes for their parental care drive. The Disney stylization of animals is another case in point. Gould has devoted a whole article to the neoteny of Mickey Mouse.

To the slightly rounded protruding forehead and peachy cheeks of many cute girls, Guthrie would add as a neotenic trait the pink cheek spots in some women. Pink cheeks are associated with youth and vigor. Those who do not come by them naturally often employ rouge or other artificial embellishments to mimic their lost youth.

But to return to the "baby face": With the preference for that understandable liking often went a preference for the baby voice. "Betty Boop" epitomized the type, and today there are several well known show biz ladies with all the appropriate and much admired fetal endowments—and more—plus the baby voice. Many women, especially of working-class background, retain a baby voice into old age. It seems likely that the retention of a baby voice is the product of the babying such women received from those who thought it "cute." To judge from the frequency with which such baby-voiced women appear in soap operas, movies, and TV commercials, the baby voice has a wide appeal for women as well as men. The baby voice, it would appear, constitutes an artificially maintained neotenous or infantilized trait when it occurs in adult women. What lies behind its attraction seems to be a combination of factors consisting primarily of

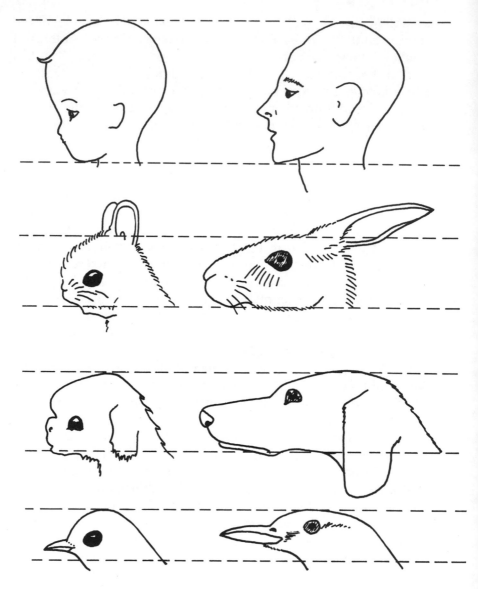

Fig. 11. The tendency to respond with cuddly and caring behavior to rounded, stubby features and relatively large eyes: *left:* child, jerboa, Pekinese dog, robin; *right:* man, hare, hound, golden oriole. (After Lorenz)

a response to the appeal of the dependent infant—its cuteness, weakness, vulnerability, and need to be protected—together with the feeling of power it gives those who speak with an adult voice. The baby voice is a ritualized appeasing, nonthreatening behavior. It is akin to the compelling nature of the infant's cry, which exerts a force difficult to resist. It may be that the higher-pitched voice of the female also represents a neotenous trait. Fascinating here, too, is the fact that babies are much more responsive to high-pitched than to low-pitched voices, and that mothers especially, and others quite often, spontaneously adopt high-pitched voices, without being aware of it, when talking to babies and children. It is interesting to observe also how the voice is modulated to the appropriate pitch and tone in relation to the age of the child. Grammar and vocals are similarly ad-justed.

Sexual Differences

Crook (1972) has conjectured that it is the combination of paedomorphic and secondary sexual characteristics that initially render women attractive to young—and, he might have added, older—men. Smoothness of face and body, voice tone, complexion, and girlish behavior all have a childlike quality, which, among other things, lowers the probability of any hostile masculine response. The same characteristics serve to reduce male fear and anxiety on closer approach, and to permit sexual expression. The male begins various display activities and show-off performances, from physical prowess to charm. The female may choose to respond or reject them. Closer approach to the muscularly more powerful male is likely to be alarming, so the male switches to his childish forms of behavior: playfulness, teasing, self-mockery, smiles, and laughter, and above all, to contact tenderness. As Crook says, "Such childlike behavior seems highly likely to stimulate not only a reciprocal sexual tenderness but also maternal aspects of the female care-giving behavior."

The female, as in virtually all other traits, is more paedomorphic than the male, and in some groups, such as Mongoloids, the sexual difference is even more marked than it is among Negroids and Caucasoids. Mongoloid women accordingly tend to be more paedomorphic than women of other groups. Not only do women of Mongoloid origin present more prominent and rounded foreheads, but the bones of the whole skull, and, indeed, the whole skeleton, are more delicately made. Mongoloids generally tend to be shorter, and have larger heads, including larger brains—150 cc by volume greater, on the average, than Caucasoids. The face is flatter, the jaws and palate smaller, the nose smaller and flatter at the root (the miscalled "bridge"), and the slight fold of skin over the median part of the eye (the epicanthic fold) is preserved. The body is less hirsute, and there are fewer hairs per square centimeter to the scalp. All these are fetal traits. One result of this is the high frequency of beauty among Mongoloid males and females, a beauty of great delicacy (see Table I, page 21).

The differential action of neoteny has produced some peculiar effects. For example, among the highly neotenized Japanese the male upper and lower jaws have been reduced in size while the teeth have not. The result has created a disharmony in many males in the form of extreme crowding and malocclusion of the teeth. This seems not, however, to compromise the physical well-being of those so affected.

Cranial Sutures

Another neotenous feature of great interest is the manner in which the sutures of the human skull, in accommodation to the growth of the brain and the eruption of the milk and permanent teeth, remain open well into the third decade. During the latter period they begin to undergo closure (see Figure 10, page 27). In apes the cranial sutures commence bony union (synostosis) during early childhood. The one exception to this rule is the premaxillary suture, which in development separates the maxillary and premaxillary bones. The premaxilla lodges the upper incisor teeth; all the other teeth are lodged in the maxilla. The premaxillary suture remains open on each side of the facial aspect of the upper jaw in the apes into adult life, whereas in humans it is obliterated by fusion of the maxilla with the premaxilla by about the tenth week of fetal life. The extremely early closure of the facial premaxillary suture is the result of the neotenous reduction of the face and upper jaw in humans; hence it is to be regarded as a neotenous feature peculiar to humans. The fusion of the premaxilla with the maxilla acts as a brake upon the forward growth of the upper jaw (prognathism) so characteristic of monkeys and apes. The palatine portion of the premaxilla and its suture remain open late into adult life (Figure 12).

Since the growth of the brain is not completed until the end of the twentieth year, the cranial sutures must remain open until

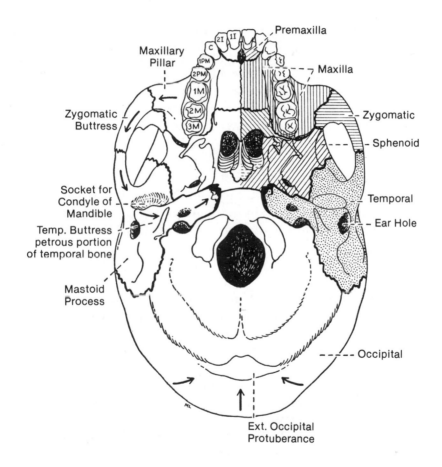

Fig. 12. Showing the palatine portion of the premaxilla. The numbers on the teeth refer to incisors, canines, premolars, and molars.

then at the very least. In fact, they do not begin to undergo
obliteration till the end of the twenty-seventh year. Occasionally,
owing to some abnormal cause, the sutures unite in early childhood and prevent the brain from increasing in size—a condition
known as microcephaly; children in whom this occurs are mentally retarded all their lives. The major and fundamental part of
human learning occurs during the first five years of life, and, as
may be seen from Table V, it is during this period that the greater
part of brain growth occurs.

The Brain

Since Bolk's day we have acquired a great deal of knowledge
concerning the growth of the human brain, all of which is in
accord with the views he expressed. The rapid rate of growth of
the human brain during the first few years of life preserves something of the rapid growth rate during fetal development. The
achievement of its ultimate great size is clearly a neotenous trait.
Detailed discussion of the brain may be deferred to the next
chapter. Here we may note that during fetal development, from
the end of embryonic age to birth, body weight increases on the
average for both sexes approximately 700 percent, and brain
weight almost as much, to wit, 540 percent. The body attains
about 5 percent of its mature weight *in utero,* and 95 percent
during postnatal growth of some twenty or more years. This is a
very slow rate of growth and may be regarded as a neotenous
trait. Physical development during infancy is rapid. Infants increase almost 50 percent in length and almost 300 percent in
weight during the first year, and about half that rate during the
second year. After that, growth slows down till it ceases in post-
adolescence.

Increase in brain size has been a striking factor in the evolution of the human species, although within the normal range of
variability there is no relationship between brain size and intelligence. As a neotenous feature the large size of the human brain is
interesting in many respects. Instead of continuing to increase in
size the brain has increased in surface area, by deepening of the
fissures between the folds or convolutions. Here, too, the sexual

---

TABLE V
Growth of the Human Brain

Fetus Lunar Months[a]	Weight (g)	Gain (g)	Percentage of Gain	
5	62.5	25.5	40.0	
6	88.0	25.5	29.0	
8	277.0	189.0	68.6	A threefold increase in weight in this two-month period.
9 birth	350/392	73/115	29.3	An increment of about a third the previous month's weight.
½ year	656.0	306.0	46.7	Almost doubles in weight in first six months.
1	825.0	169.0	20.5	Reduction to half rate of increase of first six months.
2	1,010.0	185.0	18.3	Reduction to half rate of increase of first six months.
3	1,115.0	105.0	9.4	Reduction to one-third rate of increase of first six months.
4	1,180.0	75.0	6.4	Gradual deceleration of rate of growth.
6	1,250.0	70.0	5.6	
9	1,307.0	57.0	4.3	
12	1,338.0	31.0	2.3	
20–29	1,396.0	58.0	4.1	

[a] Lunar month = 29½ days.

differences are interesting. Despite the fact that the absolute dimensions of the body and brain are smaller in girls than in boys, their intrauterine rate of growth is the same as that of boys, and the weight and size of the brain is about the same. However, in the female, brain weight in adolescent and adult is $2\frac{1}{2}$ percent of body weight as compared with 2 percent in the male. So in relative brain weight the female is neotenously ahead of the male.

While in some traits the rate of development has been accelerated, in most others development has been retarded; that is, it has occurred at a slower pace and/or extended over a greater period of time. In the evolution of the primates there has been a progressive tendency toward increase in body size as well as a prolongation of all stages of development. The adult gorilla alone among primates exceeds the human in weight. Humans, however, are characterized by heavier weight at birth. The duration of pregnancy in apes is much the same as it is in humans, differing, if at all, by being a few weeks longer in humans. The same holds true for the duration of each intrauterine developmental period. However, after birth all developmental periods—infancy, childhood, adolescence, and adulthood—are greatly extended in humans as compared with apes. In the female ape, menarche (the first menstruation) occurs at about eight years of age, whereas in humans it appears at about thirteen years in civilized societies and later in nonliterate and economically disadvantaged ones. The gradual process of sexual development between menarche and the ability to reproduce is characterized by anovulatory menstrual cycles. This is known as the adolescent sterility period. In the chimpanzee, the only ape for which we have good data, the adolescent sterility interval averages about fifteen months. In the human female the adolescent sterility interval lasts, on the average, about three years. There is, however, a great deal of variability; some females, among both apes and humans, commence to ovulate more or less regularly from the first menstrual cycle, but most do not.

Not only is gestation longer in humans than in apes, but so is the period of labor. Unlike all other primate mothers, human mothers do not lick their infants. Labor is prolonged in humans, in order, it may be conjectured, that the baby may receive adequate cutaneous stimulation from the contracting uterus. Such stimulation of the skin (and the skin is really the external nervous system of the body) serves to activate the infant's genitourinary and gastrointestinal tracts, as well as the respiratory tract. In all primates with the exception of humans this is achieved by licking; in humans it is achieved by the process of labor.

Bolk

One of the difficulties with Bolk's discussion of neoteny lay in the emphasis he placed on fetalization. This led him to perceive neoteny as working by the preservation of fetal stages of development into adult life, and to focus therefore largely on bodily traits. In his concentration on fetalization Bolk failed to perceive the clear behavioral consequences of paedomorphism. Nevertheless he did see that many bodily features in which humans resembled apes were to some extent present in the fetuses and infants of apes. He also saw that while in the apes these features represent transitional stages of development and disappear, in humans these stages become permanent. It is for this reason, as Bolk pointed out, that the fetuses of monkeys and the infants of apes look so very much like humans—not because they are descended from human-looking ancestors but because humans have retained these fetal traits in their own development. Unlike humans the apes go on to further development by an opposite principle, namely, the development in the adult of traits that were adult in their ancestral forms. This process, as we have already had occasion to observe, was termed *gerontomorphism* by de Beer (1930).

In humans the reproductive system matures in adolescence while the body remains neotenously juvenile, whereas in apes both the reproductive system and the body develop ancestral traits at an accelerated rate. As Bolk put it, adult humans in many of their traits are sexually mature fetuses. Humans have retained the fetal and youthful features of their ancestors, but apes have not.

As de Beer has shown, paedomorphosis is capable of producing large changes in the evolution of animals without loss of flexibility, whereas gerontomorphosis is incapable of this. The earlier a trait appears in individual development (ontogeny) the more extended is the time available for its development. The reason a paedomorphic species is likely to be characterized by a greater degree of evolutionary flexibility is, first, because it is probably endowed with many more new genes than the old species, and, second, because the range of individual variation is likely to be greater—two conditions which make for greater adaptive flexibility. The flexibility applies not merely at the species level but also at the level of the individual organism.

BOLK ON RACIAL DIFFERENTIATION

In 1929 Bolk put himself on record with regard to racial differentiation. In earlier writings he had referred to fetalization and retardation as important factors in the differentiation of human races, but had never developed his views at length. He now did so in the *American Journal of Physical Anthropology*.

Bolk seems to have had some difficulty in understanding Darwin, for he commences with the statement that Darwinian and Lamarckian theories are insufficient to explain the origin of new species. With respect to Lamarck he was, of course, right, but quite wrong in respect to Darwin. Darwin's theory of natural selection is, as a general principle, sufficient to explain the origin of species, with the proviso that not all naturally selected changes are necessarily of adaptive value, nor all those of adaptive value necessarily selected. Bolk felt that the origin of new species was more likely to be due to the action of internal factors. In this he was much influenced by Sir Arthur Keith's presidential address to the anthropological section of the British Association for the Advancement of Science in 1919. From this Bolk quotes the following: "The bodily and mental features which mark the various races of mankind are best explained by the theory, that the conformation of man (and ape and every vertebrate animal) is determined by a common growth controlling mechanism which is resident in a system of small but complex glandular organs." Bolk quotes other writers who went much further than Keith in attributing various effects to endocrine glands—the glands of internal secretion. For example, Bolk quotes from an article entitled "The Relation Between Racial and Constitutional Investigations" (1923) by Pfuhl, who wrote that "Each race is characterized by a type of hormonic equilibrium of its own, by which it is essentially different from all other races. The entity of somatic and mental properties of a race depends on the action of its endocrine system. All constitutional differences between the human races are manifestations of the differences of the hormonic equilibrium," and further, "Somatic features as such are not objects of inheritance, but special functional faculties of the organs transmitted." Bolk cites other writers to the same effect.

In fairness to Bolk it should be said that this was the period, in the Twenties, when the functions of the endocrine glands were really first being discovered, and as is not infrequently the case, the revelation of their striking effects in both health and disease was accompanied by somewhat exaggerated claims for what they could do. This was the day of Dr. Steinach's "monkey glands," the grafting of which into aged men, it was claimed, would restore the jaded remnants of their effete virility to full potency and possibly youth. This was the period of such bestselling books as Dr. Louis Berman's *The Glands Regulating Personality* (1921/35), in which the author endeavored to demonstrate what the title of his book suggested. Bolk makes reference to an article by the American anatomist Charles Stockard, in which views similar to his own were expressed. These views were later to be developed by Stockard in his book *The Physical Basis of Personality* (1931), and in his eight-hundred-page posthumously published monograph, *The Genetic and Endocrine Basis for Differences in Form and Behavior* (1941). Bolk, however, states that while individual characteristics, common family features, and racial traits are manifestations of the action of hormones, it is not of primary importance to show that the formation of races is due to such action, "but that the nature of racial characteristics is in accordance with the evolutionary principle of our theory, *i.e.,* that they are effects of a retarded development."

Bolk drew attention to the findings of Muller that the Malayans of Java have much smaller thyroid glands than do Caucasoids, and that the pituitary gland is heavier in Caucasoids than in Malaysians. A similar difference exists between Chinese and Caucasoids. Anatomist J. Shellshear also found that the thymus gland, situated at the front of the neck and passing into the upper part of the chest, persists among the Chinese, sometimes into old age. Shellshear regarded the persistence of the thymus as an expression of retarded development, a more general evidence of which he saw in the neotenous "childlike" appearance of the Chinese—a view with which both Keith and Bolk were in full agreement.

In recent years investigations of the thymus gland have revealed that it secretes a number of hormones, among them a growth-promoting substance called promine. Dr. Albert Szent-Gyorgi has shown that the thymus reaches its peak when growth of the body is fastest. In his studies on bovines, Szent-Gyorgi found that the thymus is somehow connected with youth, and that extracts injected into old animals make them behave as young ones. In this respect, he stated, promine is similar in its action to the "juvenile hormone," also known as the "Peter Pan hormone," found in insects that undergo metamorphosis into butterflies.

In addition to producing a large number of lymphocytes, the thymus also produces a variety of hormones and plays an important role in the development of immunologic competence in fetus and child. There is also good evidence that maturation of fetal liver and splenic cells is dependent on an intact thymus. Removal of the thymus in newborn mice stunts their growth; thymus-derived serum (gamma globulin) injected into such animals causes them to grow faster, to maintain a higher weight average, and survive almost twice as long as thymectomized controls who have been given a neutral serum.

The thymus grows rapidly throughout the fetal period and reaches its maximum size in relation to body weight at birth. After birth, slower growth continues until puberty, after which much of its substance is replaced by fatty tissue.

Juvenile hormone has been found in high concentration in the thymus of all mammals thus far investigated. It may well turn out that promine or some other substance produced by the thymus, the timing of which is genetically regulated, is the hormone or one of the hormones of neoteny.

Bolk suggested that differentiation of the races of *Homo sapiens* was due to differences in rates of retardation. "In the groups subjected to the more effective retardation, conditions will persist in a stage of development which is passed by the other groups continuing their development till a farther point.'' If this view is correct, Bolk argued, then it would be necessary to show that the somatic differences between the races are phenomena of fetalization. If the formation of races is due to differences in retardation, those races that have been least fetalized will also be least retarded in the physiological sense; their vital course will be quicker, the duration of their life shorter. This Bolk blithely proceeded to demonstrate to his satisfaction, if not to that of most of his contemporary fellow-scientists. Some sixty years later Bolk's main claim does not appear to be as extreme as it once seemed. Unfortunately, the examples he chose to support his argument were open to serious question; for example, Bolk found that American blacks in 1920 lived, on the average, some fifteen years less than whites. This great disparity he believed could not be accounted for on environmental grounds. But contrary to what Bolk believed, the evidence that has become available since he wrote shows beyond dispute that environmental conditions, indeed, make all the difference between black and white mortality rates. With the improvement, such as it has been, in living conditions for blacks generally, the expectation of life at birth has increased, and the differences in life expectancy between blacks and whites have progressively decreased. Bolk quotes the figures for 1920. I also give here the figures for 1978.

EXPECTATION OF LIFE AT BIRTH

Year	White Females	Black Females	White Males	Black Males
1920	56.41	42.35	54.05	40.45
1978	77.7	73.7	70.2	65.3

Source: *Vital Statistics Report,* U.S. Dept of HEW, August 13, 1979.

These figures are striking and speak for themselves. In 1920 black women had an expectation of life that was fourteen years less than that of white women. That difference in 1978 was reduced to four years, and their longevity had increased by thirty-one years! The figures are pretty much the same for the differences in expectation of life for black as compared with white males. In short, the difference in life expectancy between blacks and whites has been reduced from fourteen years in 1920 for both sexes to four years in 1978 in females and somewhat less than five years in males. There can be little doubt that with further (much overdue) improvements in the socioeconomic conditions of blacks, the differences will be reduced to the vanishing point.

Bolk complained in 1929 of our lack of knowledge concerning the development of physiological traits among the different populations of humanity. That complaint is still justified. Nevertheless, we have good data for several such traits, including the onset of menstruation, menarche. Age of menarche varies from fourteen to seventeen years among different African peoples, but in New York City black and white girls of similar socioeconomic background, menarche apppears at the same average age, about twelve and a half years. When Japanese immigrants into America give birth and raise children in their new homeland, the new Americans grow to be taller than their cousins who have remained in Japan. Indeed, all the evidence we have—such as it is—relating to the development of physiological traits among the different varieties of humankind indicates that under similar socioeconomic and physiographic conditions they would develop in much the same way.

TEETH AND BRACHYCEPHALIZATION

Bolk cites rates of growth and eruption of the teeth, which are somewhat more rapid in blacks than in whites, as evidence of the greater retardation of the latter. He also cites skin color as a fetal trait that has persisted in whites, unlike blacks in whom it becomes more or less deeply pigmented shortly after birth. Since a relatively pigmentless skin is a fetal trait, Bolk appears to be here on sound enough ground. Fortunately, however, for the human species, which underwent almost the whole of its evolution in Africa in areas of high sunlight intensity, all babies developed the ancestral skin color of their ancestors, all of whose skins were pigmented. In such high sunlight intensity environments, pigmented skin has many adaptive advantages over a white skin: it does not burn as easily, nor as readily develop cancer, under such conditions as white skin does; it serves to keep the body cool by more efficient sweating. As good a case, or even better, could be made for pigmented skin's being neotenous for its ecological setting as could be made for "white" skin as neotenous for its own setting. It all depends upon the ethnocentric distorting-glass through which one happens to be looking.

Brachycephaly—that is, broadheadedness—in contrast to dolichocephaly (longheadedness) also appears to be a fetal trait. Up to the sixth fetal month the head tends to be long. The "brachycephalic races," Bolk suggested, are the offspring of longheaded ones. In the course of time, he argued, the transforming processes in some groups of humanity were retarded and, growing weaker, "the initial fetal form of the skull was increasingly retained," until, finally, brachycephaly was established as the persisting form of the head. After the sixth month the fetal cephalic (head) index varies from mesocephalic 75.9 to 79.9, to brachycephalic 80.0 to 84.9.

A study of the brachycephalization of recent mankind, published by distinguished anatomist and physical anthropologist Franz Weidenreich in 1945, attributed broadheadedness to the adoption of the erect posture. This is a rather dubious claim since the interiors of the skulls of apes are broad (brachycephalic), as are the cranial cavities of the australopithecines. Bolk's fetalization hypothesis makes more sense.

In the occasional failure of development of the upper lateral incisor teeth, of the upper and lower third molars, which may be either completely missing or malformed, and other similar features of the dentition, Bolk also perceives the process of retardation at work. This may be so, but another explanation is available.

With the trend toward reduction in the projection of the jaws (orthognathy) in whites, and in some Mongoloids such as the Japanese, there is a reduction of the premaxilla. The premaxilla lodges the upper central and lateral incisors. Reduced projection of the jaw comes about from the failure of the lateral portions of the premaxilla to develop, and the suppression of the *anlage* or cellular precursors for the lateral incisor. The same thing may happen at the back of the jaws. This may, of course, be seen as a form of retardation, but it is a question whether it contributes anything to the understanding of the factors involved in the variability of the human dentition.

Finally, Bolk asks: Which of the human races are most strongly fetalized? "This question is of great importance," he states, "from an anthropological as well as from a sociological point of view. For it need hardly be emphasized that a different degree of fetalization means a more or less advanced state of hominization. The further a race has been somatically fetalized and physiologically retarded, the further it has grown away from the pithecoid ancestor of man. Quantitative differences in fetalization and retardation are the base of racial unequivalence. Looked at from this point of view the division of mankind into higher and lower races is fully justified."

Bolk believed that hominization or fetalization had proceeded furthest in the "white races" as compared with the black. According to Bolk the lesser fetalization and less extended retardation is exhibited by the "black races" in their long skull, black skin, strong prognathism, more "primitive" dentition, narrower hands and feet, and more rapid development.

Bolk seems to have overlooked the fact that black peoples exhibit many fetal traits that do not occur in whites, especially those resulting from retardative growth—for example, such traits as hairlessness, nose flatness, flat root of nose, small ears, later closure of premaxillary sutures, longer eyelashes, frontal eminences, and a good many other traits as shown in Table I.

Bolk backed down from his earlier statement that the Mongoloid peoples appeared to be the most highly fetalized. In his 1929 article he stated that comparisons between Mongoloids and Europeans hardly enable one to speak of different degrees of fetalization as between the two groups; rather, each with its special traits points to a divergence in the development of fetal traits—the Europeans with light-pigmented skin, hair, and eyes, and taller stature, and the Mongoloids with the epicanthic fold, flattened bridge of the nose, stocky build, exophthalmos (pop eyes), and the fetal features of the brain. In this latter connection Bolk refers to a study by Ariens Kappers, distinguished Dutch neuroanatomist, in which he drew attention to such fetal characters of the Mongoloid brain as greater height indices, longer orbital rostrum, more rounded temporal lobes, and the general morphology of the brain. Ariens Kappers felt that such features were best explained by Bolk's fetalization theory. Bolk, however, seemed reluctant to yield pride of place in what he conceived to be the hierarchy of races, for in commenting on his colleague's study he said it would be a mistake to compare the value of these differences as evidence of a higher or lower degree of hominization. This statement would appear to be in flat contradiction to his earlier one on the preceding page that a different degree of fetalization means a more or less advanced stage of hominization. What Bolk seems to mean is that on the basis of different fetal traits exhibited by Mongoloids and Europeans there exist no grounds for assigning one to a lower degree of hominization than the other—a very generous conclusion on his part, seeing that Mongoloids outnumber "Europeans" in neotenous traits!

The terms "higher" and "lower" employed by Bolk were the current usage of his day. In "the Scale of Nature," another phrase of his day held over from the eighteenth century, animals and races were seen to be ascending the ladder of Nature in order of their progressive advancement as well as merit. It was an unfortunate usage as we may judge in retrospect, but for its time it faithfully reflected the naturalistic and sociopolitical outlook of most writers on the subject.

"Finally," wrote Bolk, "it is not superfluous to call to mind that the sociological and cultural importance of a race is not determined in the first place by its somatic, but by its psychological properties." Bolk, however, chose to leave further discussion of such matters to others more competent in that area than he.

It is, of course, unsound to speak of the "cultural and sociological importance of a race," since as human beings the members of all races are equally important culturally and sociologically, no matter what their state of technological development. Anthropologists are generally agreed that as a consequence of the unique evolutionary development of our humankind over a period of some five million years or so, during which our ancestors lived by food-gathering and hunting, and during which the challenges of the environment and the responses made to them were everywhere much the same, it would be expected that the human mind, allowing for variation in individuals within each group, is in all human "races" much the same.

Breast and Lips

One of the consequences of the prolonged immaturity and dependency of the human infant is that it necessitates a rather long nursing period, not longer than in apes who nurse their young for four or more years, but seemingly long for so active a species as *Homo sapiens*. In adaptation to the erect posture and the shrinkage of the jaws, there has been a further adaptive response in the development of hemispherical breasts in the female, and the unique response to this in the form of everted mucous-membranous lips in humans. Such everted lips are much better adapted to suckling at a hemispherical surface than are the thin lips of apes. Just as the cheeks of the baby with their suctorial pads of fat are very different from those of the later child and the adult, so does the character of the lips differ in the baby from what they will later become in child and adult. The newborn baby's lips are characterized by small papillae, and a large median papilla on the upper lip, which enable the baby to secure a firmer grip on the areolar region of the breast, and to convert his mouth into an hermetically sealed oral suction pump. The nipple lies between tongue and palate. The baby does not suck the nipple; were he to do so he would produce a partial vacuum in his mouth and fail to develop the ability to suckle properly. The highly sensitive vascularized spongy lips of the baby are beautifully designed to do a great number of things at the breast: the first is to milk it by suckling (*not* sucking—a very different thing); the second is to send all sorts of messages to the mother, psychological as well as physiological, which produce an interchange between mother and infant having a fundamental effect upon the development of both. The effect is not only physiological but also human, for it is at the breast that the beginning humanization of the child commences. More than four hundred years ago William Painter wrote of the breast as "that most sacred fountaine of the body, the educatour of mankind"—a statement fully supported by everything we have since learned. In short, what happens between mother and infant in the breastfeeding situation, from the first few minutes following birth and thereafter, constitutes the foundational experiences upon which human behavioral capacities are optimally developed. It is within the first few hours that the primary bonding occurs; this can happen only when mother and infant are in contact, and will best transpire when the baby is put to nurse. at the mother's breast. The physiological and psychological benefits that mother and infant, in all mammals, reciprocally confer upon each other during that interchange are so fundamental, it is evident that they were designed to continue in this manner the symbiotic relationship they had maintained throughout the uterogestative period. The extended nature of this relationship may perhaps be interpreted as a neotenous phenomenon, in the sense that it represents a continuation of the uterogestative relationship.

We shall have something more to say on the importance and nature of breastfeeding in the next chapter.

Hairlessness

Humans are characterized by a relative hairlessness (glabrousness) that stands in marked contrast to the thick pelage that covers the bodies of other primates, especially the great apes. Plato (not seriously) defined man as a featherless biped. In response to this, Diogenes plucked a fowl and presented it as Plato's man. Others have designated our species the naked ape and similar defamatory names. But humans are neither naked nor apes. Humans in fact have quite as many hairs as apes. Except on the head, the hair in humans doesn't grow as long as it does in apes. The retardation or reduction of body hair in humans almost certainly followed upon the adoption of the erect posture and a new way of life, resulting in certain physiological changes that favored the perpetuation of genotypes (genetic constitutions) for reduced hair. It also appears to have been of advantage for hair to remain and even to increase in density on certain parts of the body, such as the head, eyebrows, face, pubic and perineal regions, and armpits. In what manner could such adaptive changes have been brought about?

It has been suggested that the answer may be provided by the hunting way of life, in which humans spent almost the whole of their evolutionary history. In hunting much running is necessary, and the chase may extend over hours or even days. Under such conditions in a torrid environment, the body will become heated. Overheating is dangerous and can be lethal. That humans were originally tropical animals is indicated, among other things, by the fact that their normal body temperature is 98.6° Fahrenheit. Humans tolerate heat better than cold, and by the use of culturally developed devices are capable of living under all climatic conditions, from the pole of cold to the summers of Philadelphia.

The new hunting way of life meant that some means of eliminating the body heat generated during the hunt was vitally necessary. Even more important was the development of some mechanism by which the body could be protected against heat accumulation, and not merely as an emergency device for its elimination. This is most effectively achieved by sweating. Forest-dwelling animals generally do not possess sweat glands; the air by which they are surrounded is heavily saturated with moisture, and this, together with their habit of avoiding overheating and prolonged exposure to heat, is more than adequate to protect them against its effects. The great apes, for example, normally proceed about their activities at a leisurely pace, and spend much of their time in the shade, at rest or in sleep. Sweat glands in apes are not well developed. The gorilla, the chimpanzee, and to a lesser extent the orangutan possess a mixture of both ordinary (eccrine) and specialized (apocrine) glands in their armpits. Humans, on the other hand, possess the largest number of sweat glands of any animal, and there is no other animal that exhibits so speedy a sweat response. Usually, on a hot day, the only animals likely to be seen sweating at the zoo are the visitors outside the animal enclosures. The rhinoceros, the hippopotamus, and elephant are also relatively hairless, and when they run hard and overheat they sweat, but unlike humans they are well insulated with a layer of fat and do not normally either hunt (since they are herbivores) or get overheated. Humans sweat from almost every part of their body surfaces. Caucasoids and American blacks have about 750 sweat glands to each square inch of skin. African blacks have more sweat glands than other peoples. Mongoloids have about 450 sweat glands per square inch. Since fetus and infant have fewer sweat glands than adults, Mongoloids are more neotenous in this respect than other peoples.

It was the hunting way of life that almost certainly resulted in the development in humans of the largest number of sweat glands to be found in any animal, a system of glands capable of producing two quarts of sweat per hour over the body surface! This would amount to the removal of twelve hundred calories per hour from the body, and a reduction of body heat by 68° Fahrenheit. Body thermoregulation could hardly be more efficiently achieved. As Professor Yas Kuno writes, "The maximal rate of sweating seems to be that required to maintain constancy of body temperature in outdoor life under hot sunshine." The gathering-hunting way of life is incompatible with a heavy growth of body hair, and principally because of this incompatibility, it is likely that humans became the only relatively hairless members of the primates, hair of some density being retained only where it served an adaptively useful purpose.

Against this theory it has been argued that other hunting animals have not lost their fur. This is true, but other animals are high-speed, short-chase hunters who do not pursue their prey for hours or even days, as contemporary hunting peoples often do.

The reduction of body hair and number of sweat glands has gone furthest in that major group of humans in which in every other respect the most advanced morphological developments have occurred, to wit, in the Mongoloid major group. Both in the density of hair follicles and in the actual number of hairs per square centimeter there has been an appreciable reduction.

The question has been raised as to the meaning of baldness. The answer is that we do not know. What we do know is that there are several patterns of baldness, and that therefore a number of genes must be involved that, under the influence of male hormones, result in baldness. In the absence of male hormones, as in females, baldness almost never occurs.

An alternative theory of relative human hairlessness, a sort of shortcut to the hunting-chase thermoregulation theory, holds that human hairlessness is simply due to a mutation. This is quite possible, for mutations do not tend to survive unless they have some adaptive value. It is not enough, however, to speak of "neotenous mutations." The mutant genes must pass through the sieve of natural selection before the traits they affect can become established in a population.

Elliot Smith failed to perceive that this was almost exactly

To account for the loss of body hair, Desmond Morris has suggested that the naked body would be reciprocally more attractive in sexual signaling, but that sensitivity to touch was probably sexually most important. In sexual encounters both male and female would become more highly sensitized to erotic stimuli. In a species in which pair-bonding was evolving, this would heighten the pleasure of sexual excitement and contribute to the bonding of the pair by intensifying copulatory rewards. With neoteny to help the process on its way, Morris adds, hairlessness would become a viable proposition.

There have also been theories offered to complement the theory of the protective function of hair where it has not been reduced but has thickened on the human body. One such theory holds that the hair in these regions serves a sexually selective purpose. The various striking elaborations of hair colors, hair tufts, mustaches, beards, capes, and the like, in many monkeys, suggests the possibility of sexual selection. In humans, hair distribution may to some extent have served a similar purpose.

Regarding the variety of eye and hair colors encountered among humans, McConnaill and Ralphs have shown that there is good reason to believe that the basic eye and hair colors were dark blue eyes and blond hair. If that is so, these investigators argue, then "the mutation that gave rise to the retention by the adult of blue eyes and light blond hair is to be reckoned as a change leading to the retention of an infantile characteristic: it is paedomorphic, and therefore, formally progressive. It is comparable in this respect with thickness of lip and hairlessness of the body."

There is much else to be said on the subject of hair, for in addition to its protective and attractional functions hair has many others, such as the roles it plays in the diffusion of odors, and in determining age-grading, status, and venerability. Graying of back hair in the gorilla is associated with age and leadership. Graying of the head hair in humans is, in many cultures, similarly evaluated. The different styles of hair in infrahuman primates and those adopted by men and women undoubtedly serve a sexual function. Since it has been claimed that bald-headed men tend to be more sexually virile than hairy-headed men, it may be that sexual selection—that is, the preference of some women for bald-headed men because of their putative virility—has played a role in the distribution of the gene in some societies and not in others. It is possible, then, that in the distribution of the varieties of hair form encountered in humans—frizzy, tightly coiled, wavy, and straight—and in its various coloration, sexual selection may have played a significant role.

It would seem reasonably clear, then, that the mechanisms through which the selective advantages of relative hairlessness of the human body were brought about, as well as the various other characteristics of hair, were mainly, if not entirely, the result of neoteny.

Giving Bolk His Due

Not everyone was enamored of Bolk's fetalization theory. Grafton Elliot Smith (1927), the British anatomist, thought little of Bolk's attempt to explain the emergence of the distinctive human traits as due to the restraining influence of the endocrine glands. "Man," Elliot Smith asserted, "is not simply a simian infant! The great distinctive feature of the Human Family is an enormous active growth and development of the brain and the profound transformation of its mental powers, which are left unexplained by Bolk's speculation."

Clearly Elliot Smith failed to understand what Bolk was saying, as he apparently failed to understand what Keith had been saying even before Bolk. Yet, fifteen pages earlier in the same book, Elliot Smith wrote,

> The retention of primitive characters is often to be looked upon as a token that their possessor has not been compelled to turn aside from the straight path and adopt protective specializations, but has been able to preserve some of the plasticity associated with his primitiveness, precisely because he has not succumbed or fallen away in the struggle for supremacy. It is the wider triumph of the individual who specializes late, after benefitting by the many-sided experience of early life, over him who in youth becomes tied to one narrow calling.
>
> In many respects Man retains more of the primitive characteristics —for example, in his hands—than his nearest simian relatives.

what Bolk was saying, the very phenomenon for which at the same time he was attempting to provide an evolutionary mechanism.

Bolk attempted to claim too much for neoteny as a factor in the evolution of humankind, as if the development of all human physical traits were due to neotenous processes. In claiming too much he exhibited the common failing of those who become so enamored of a theory that they become insensible to the facts that happen not to agree with it. The truth is that there have been many changes in human evolution that were not due to neoteny, such as the overbite (the upper front teeth biting over the lower), the erect posture, the relative proportion of the limbs to each other and to the body, buttocks, head hair, baldness, and the large penis.

Ernst Mayr, the Harvard zoologist, has described Bolk's fetalization hypothesis as a misleading theory. The theory, he writes, "that the hominid line has passed through a gorilla-orang stage and has since become 'fetalized' is not supported by the known facts."

But "the known facts" today have rendered that statement more than debatable. The evidence of amino acid and protein analysis indicates that the genome (the total number of genes of each type) differences between the great apes and humans is no more than that which exists between sibling species, approximately 1 percent. As already mentioned, it may well be that the gene changes accounting for physical differences between human and chimpanzee represent a small fraction of that 1 percent, involving primarily changes in gene regulation rather than structural genes. Substantial differences in gene regulation would be sufficient to account for both the physical and behavioral differences between ape and human.

As for the statement that the hominid line has never passed through an apelike stage such as the gorilla-orang type, that may be, but as we have noted, a good candidate for such an ancestor is a form very like the pygmy chimpanzee. With respect to fetalization, whatever it may have been in the mind of Bolk or some other writers, it is not here being claimed that either fetalization, neoteny, or paedomorphosis was the sole factor in the evolution of humankind; rather, they have been major factors—important, neglected, slighted, denied, and not understood. It is our claim here that a fuller understanding of the role that neoteny or paedomorphosis has played in the evolution of humanity would greatly contribute to our understanding of that past history and the role it should be playing in the direction of our future individual and social development.

"The brain," Mayr has written, "is ahead in ontogeny in all mammals. Indeed, since human babies have extremely large brains, one might say exactly the opposite of what Bolk has said and state that they have become 'adultified.' " This, however, is to misinterpret the facts, as reference to Table V (p. 43) will at once show. It will be seen from that table that it is not so much babies who have extremely large brains, but seven- to nine-month-old fetuses. The most rapid growth of the human brain occurs from the end of the sixth fetal month to the end of the ninth fetal month, and although the rate of growth is somewhat reduced after birth it is nevertheless quite considerable well into the third year. It is *this early rapid rate of brain growth* from the end of the sixth fetal month into the third year that is neotenous.

The unfavorable criticism that Bolk's ideas have sometimes received has not always been just; that criticism for the most part has been ably disposed of by Gould. Where Bolk may be faulted is in his anti-Darwinism, in his own antiquated theory of evolution, in his belief that hormones are the principal agents of paedomorphosis, and in his view that virtually all human traits can be explained by fetalization. Except for the notion that so-called "racial" differences have been mainly produced by neoteny, Bolk's ideas on the subject of race and the conclusions he draws from those erroneous ideas are wholly unsound. However, Bolk's main idea, that it is to the slow progress of our life's course that we owe our human traits, remains an enduring contribution to our better understanding of the mechanism of human evolution.

2

Neoteny and the Evolution of Human Behavior

If it can be shown that behavioral neoteny is a
generalized human trait, an important conceptual
advance will have been made toward understanding
many of the distinctive attributes of man.
— WILLIAM MASON

The neotene who marches upright
— W. H. AUDEN
Grub first, then ethics

We have seen that the stages of physical and physiological development in the evolution of humankind have been greatly extended in *Homo sapiens* as compared with our forerunners, and
most significantly as compared with our nearest relations, the
great apes. What has hitherto been neglected in discussions of
neoteny has been the role it has played in the development of
human behavior.

The capacity for learning is characteristic of the juvenile ape,
to a comparatively limited extent, and to a much greater extent
of the human infant and child. We see this most strikingly in the
retention and development of the ability to play, the sense of
humor, the ability to learn, the continuing growth and development of curiosity and inventiveness, and the remarkable uses of
the imagination, the ability to make believe, traits that juvenile

apes exhibit to a quite marked degree, but that fail to develop as they mature.

Brain and Mind

Not many gene changes would have been necessary to produce those qualitative changes serving to differentiate the human from the ape mind. It would appear that the principal developments associated with such changes have been those facilitating complex symbol usage. What the structural nature of these changes may have been is at present conjectural. Increase in the number of cerebral neurons and in the fine connections between them, with increased capacity for growth and development, resulting in more complex circuits and in the improvement of the association, scanning, and feedback capacities of the brain, is one possibility. The late Professor Edward L. Thorndike once remarked that "in their deeper nature the higher forms of intellectual operation are identical with mere association or connection forming, depending upon the same sort of physiological connections but requiring many more of them." Certain it is, as many workers have shown, that the selection pressure making for greater development of the association areas of the brain has been greater in humans than in other primates. In the evolution of the brain, increase in size was important because increase in tissue mass was necessary for the complex variety of processing a human brain requires. Increase in brain size is to a large extent the result of increase in size in the different specialized areas. The behavior of which an animal is capable is determined more by the size of its specialized areas than by the overall size of the brain. For example, the size of the motor area of the brain that controls a particular muscle relates not to the size of the muscle but to the skill with which it is used. As the late Ralph Gerard remarked, the reason why chimpanzees will never learn to speak, in spite of our best efforts to help them do so, is probably that they don't have large enough motor areas for tongue and larynx. The human motor area for the tongue is much larger than the one for the whole leg. A cerebral area for a tail is nonexistent in the human, but in the spider monkey, with an extraordinarily prehensile tail, the tail area represented in the brain is huge.

The differences between the human and the ape brain are probably based on a very small number of gene changes, the net effect of which has been an increase in educability. Indeed, educability is the outstanding species characteristic of humans. The juvenile ape is more educable than the adult ape, and the suggestion here is that the preservation of the educability of the juvenile ape into the adult stage in humans led, by similar gene changes, to the development of the distinctively human brain.

The theory outlined here suggests that the shift from the status of ape to the status of human being was the result, in large part, of neotenous mutations having a high selective value for the retention of the growth trends of the juvenile brain and its potentialities for learning at all stages of development. It is clear that the nature of these potentialities for learning must also have undergone intrinsic change, for no amount of extension of the ape's capacity for learning would yield a human mind. The genes for it are simply not there.

Evolution of the human mental faculties by neoteny was almost certainly a gradual process. It is unlikely, though not impossible, that the shift from ape to hominid status was saltatory either for physical or mental traits. It may be doubted, for example, that *Homo erectus* was as intelligent as Neandertal man, though it is likely that he was more intelligent than any of the australopithecines. But even this is something of which we cannot be sure. The progressive increase in the volume of the brain in the fossil hominids seems to have been paralleled by a progressive increase in mental capacities. Size of brain seems to have stabilized itself in humans about thirty thousand years ago. This does not, however, mean that the spatial resources of the brain have come to an end. Increase can come about, as we have already noted, by deepening and multiplication of the number of cerebral convolutions, in this manner increasing the surface area of the brain without increasing its size. There is no reason to believe that either the quality or the duration of man's capacity for learning will not be subject to further evolution.

As we have already observed, during fetal development body weight increases for both sexes on the average approximately 700 percent, and brain weight increases an average of 540 percent. In humans the rate of growth of the brain exceeds that of any other primate. The brain grows at an extraordinarily rapid rate during fetal life, at the rate of 20,000 neurons a minute, and during the last three months it increases in weight at the rate of 2.2 milligrams a minute. During these final three months of fetal development there is an explosive increase in the size of the brain, from 88 grams (3 ounces) at the end of the sixth month to 372 grams (13 ounces) at birth, a gain of 284 grams (10 ounces), that is to say the brain more than quadruples in size. At this time the brain has achieved more than one-fourth its adult weight, and constitutes 10 percent of the entire body weight of the infant, as compared with only 2 percent in the adult. (See Table V.) It is during these last three months of intrauterine development that the brain undergoes a great burst of neuronal growth. From around birth to the end of the sixth postnatal month there is yet another burst of growth of nerve cells. At birth the infant's brain is closer to its adult state in size and development than is any other organ, and the explosive rate of growth that characterized it during the last three months of prenatal development to some extent continues throughout the first year, when the brain more than doubles to a weight of 825 grams (29 ounces), a gain of 453 grams (16 ounces). In the second year the gain is 185 grams (6½ ounces) to a weight of 1,010 grams (35½ ounces).

By the end of the third year the human child has achieved a brain weight of 1,115 grams (39 ounces), which is four-fifths the size of that of an adult, 1,396 grams (49¼ ounces).

Growth is increase in size, and development is increase in complexity. The postnatal growth of the human brain maintains the late fetal growth rate well into the third year, and under the stimulus of the socioeconomic environment, brain development proceeds at a cumulative rate. The human brain continues to develop for many years after the ape brain has ceased to do so. As Sir Arthur Keith pointed out, in this prolongation of cerebral growth and development, we see an important "if not the most important feature of human evolution—namely, the time taken to assemble and to organize the myriads of nerve cells and of nerve tracts which enter into the structure of man's brain." This process, Keith went on to add, constituted a good example of the "law" of fetalization or neoteny.

These are important points, for together with other things they help explain—as we shall see—the physical basis of the human mind. Here attention should be drawn to the fact that the most active period of growth of the human brain after birth occurs during the first three years, a period that corresponds with the foundational learning of the child, a period when many of the child's personality and other traits are acquired. This does not for a moment imply that all subsequent learning is by comparison unimportant. What it does imply is that the first three years constitute a highly sensitive period during which the child is at his most malleable, and therefore most educable. Hence, we need to give the child during that crucial period of development more informed attention.

The growth of the brain is very different from that of the rest of the body, for while the rates of growth of the infant in length and weight up to the end of the first year are similar to those of fetal body growth (Table V), this is followed by a rapid slowing of those rates, whereas the brain continues to grow at a rapid rate well into the fourth year, slowing down only thereafter.

From the end of the second year to the end of the fifth year, when the brain reaches 1,225 grams (44½ ounces), the rate of increase is about 84 grams a year. From the sixth to the twelfth year the total increment is a mere 88 grams (3 ounces), and the gain thereafter until the cessation of increase in brain mass at about age twenty years is no more than 58 grams (2 ounces); the brain by then has reached its total weight of 1,396 grams (49¼ ounces or 3 pounds).

The newborn's brain is about 28 percent of its adult size. By the end of the first year, 62 percent of total brain growth has been achieved, and by the end of the third year, 83 percent. This is a far more rapid rate of growth than occurs in any other creature of similar size. In the rhesus monkey and in the lesser ape, the gibbon, 70 percent of brain growth has been achieved by birth; the remainder of its total brain growth is completed within the first six months. In the great apes the active period of brain growth occurs during the first eleven months, and in humans during the first thirty-six months. Complete growth of the human brain is not accomplished until the end of the second decade of life or later. In childhood the body weighs five times as much as the brain. In the adult the body weighs fifty times as much as the brain.

It is evident, then, that while the rate of growth of the brain in humans is rapid in the final three months of fetal life and early childhood development, after the third year there is a marked deceleration in the rate of growth prolonged over many years—phenomena that are essentially neotenous (Table V).

Total body weight of the human newborn averages 7 pounds. In the newborn chimpanzee total body weight is on the average $4\frac{1}{3}$ pounds (1,800) grams, and brain weight is about 200 grams (7 ounces) as compared with the human newborn brain weight of 372 grams (13 ounces). In the gorilla the total body weight of the newborn is about $4\frac{3}{4}$ pounds (1,980 grams), and brain size at birth would appear to be not much more than in the chimpanzee.

Labor in the apes generally lasts not longer than two hours, as compared with an average of fourteen hours with the firstborn and an average of eight hours with the laterborn in the human female. The smaller body size of the anthropoid newborn may to some extent be related to the shorter duration of labor in the anthropoid female. However, in the human the large body size of the baby, and especially of the head, necessitates the birth of the infant while it is still able to pass through the birth canal. This, on the average, occurs $266\frac{1}{2}$ days after conception.

In the evolution of the mammals, length of gestation has generally tended to increase along with the growth and development of the brain; paralleling this have been both the tendency to produce one offspring at a time and the greater maturity of the newborn. The most striking exception to this rule is the human newborn, who has a brain weight more than double that of the ape, and a period of physiological and behavioral immaturity that far exceeds that of most other mammals.

Cerebral Function

If the cerebrum, the brain, has been neotenized, so have its behavioral capacities—always remembering that a capacity is a potentiality, as distinct from an ability, which is a trained capacity. While the fetus's behavioral responses are mostly limited to reflex acts, it is capable of learning while still in the womb, at least during the last three months. Here, too, we should bear in mind that behavior means any act of the organism. A response is distinguished from a reaction by being experience-dependent; a reaction is an automatic behavior not dependent on previous experience. For example, during the last three months a human fetus can be conditioned, that is, taught to learn, to *respond* to the signal or sign of an original stimulus to which it has been exposed simultaneously. It is this capacity for learning, which is already apparently present in the older fetus, which is so greatly extended in humans, and which renders genetic, that is to say, fixed action patterns of behavior or instincts, both unnecessary and undesirable—unnecessary because they would be useless, and undesirable because they would act like so many bunions to impede the pilgrim's progress.

In the evolution of humankind the problem-solving ability we call intelligence has been at a high selective premium, and the outstanding characteristics of intelligence are its freedom from constraint and the striving to find a solution to the problem presented. Intelligence is to a large extent based on past experience, but that past experience is itself the product of accumulated novel solutions to past problems. In humans, genetic channeling of behavior is almost completely superseded by learned responses to environmental messages. Human behavior does not proceed in predestinate grooves, which in many animals produce a fixity of instinctive reaction but which in humans are replaced by the flexibility and experimental nature of intelligence.

Instinct commonly refers to a predetermined automatic reaction to a particular stimulus, accompanied by a particular emotion. A reflex differs from an instinct in being unaccompanied by an emotion. Intelligence is commonly understood to mean the most appropriately successful response to the challenge of a particular situation. Instinct and intelligence are usually taken to be radically opposed to each other, but as Gaston Viaud has pointed out, the opposition is not so much between instinct and intelligence as between non-intelligent instinctive acts and intelligent acts, "no matter whether the latter be instinctive or else due to the loftiest considerations."

It should be mentioned here that the so-called rigidity and fixedness of instinct in animals has been greatly overstressed. Innumerable studies in recent years have shown that instincts are not only modifiable by experience, but in addition almost always involve elements of learning. Whatever the precise origins of the human capacity for educability and intelligence, the hypothesis that best accounts for the mechanism of their evolution is neoteny, the retention of the fetal-juvenile traits of plasticity, flexibility. The reference here is to instinct defined as a fixed action tendency to an organized and biologically adaptive behavior characteristic of a given species (to be distinguished from a reflex, defined as a simple automatic reaction to a stimulus).

It was John Adams who wrote, in a letter to his wife, Abigail, that "Education has made a greater difference between man and man than nature has between man and brute." That observation recognizes that while the potentialities are normally there for growth and development as a human being, they must receive the appropriate kinds of stimulation to be fulfilled. And, of course, a healthy human being, in the sense of a person functioning adequately mentally as well as physically, can only be one whose mind has been adequately stimulated, and thus caused to grow and develop. Indeed, the evidence indicates that the proper use of the mind—its adequate exercise through both thinking and feeling—is as necessary for the health of the individual and his society as is breathing. Shallow breathing—and there are always many persons who have never learned to breathe adequately and consequently suffer from all sorts of ills—is not conducive to good physical or mental health; inadequate oxygenation of the tissues interferes with their adequate functioning. But since the person as a functioning *human* being is essentially a mental creature, a creature of mind, it is vitally necessary for him to use his mind, to think *and* to feel. Humans have come a long way by increasing not only their power to think soundly, but also their power to *feel* (emotionally) soundly. Sound thinking alone is not enough; sound feeling is at least as necessary. Indeed, emotions are perhaps even more anciently the product of neoteny than is reason.

The dissociation between emotion and reason is, in fact, an artificial one, largely the contribution of Plato to the Western world; as Plato put it in a famous image, reason stands like a charioteer reining in the unruly horses, which would otherwise run away with him. Today we recognize that our emotional development is as important as is our rational development. Emotions have played a major role in evolution, as we may judge from the funerary artifacts of prehistoric humans who, like the Neandertals of Iraq, buried their dead on a bed of flowers. The funerary practices of the Neandertals indicate a belief in the existence of life after death, as well as the existence of deep feelings and emotional involvement with their fellow men and the spiritual world in which they clearly believed. They have left the evidence of what has been called by the French biologist Cuénot their "metaphysical anxiety" in their graves for us to read. Among nonliterate peoples we observe that reason and emotion are rarely if ever as frequently dissociated as they are among civilized peoples, and in many respects they seem to be so much happier and mentally healthier than most individuals are in civilized societies. What we need to understand is that emotional health is an indispensable condition of general health, and that it is a neotenous trait that requires at least as careful nurturing as does the cultivation of the ability to think soundly.

Openmindedness, receptivity to new ideas, malleability, questing, striving, questioning, seeking, critical testing and weighing of new ideas as well as old ones; wide-eyed curiosity and excitement in the enjoyment of new experiences, the willingness to work hard at making sense of it all, together with a sense of humor and laughter—all these are neotenous traits. Indeed, all these are *needs* seeking satisfaction in the opportunities for growth and development, which it should be a fundamental purpose of every society to provide.

Educability

Educability, humanity's species characteristic, is not simply a matter of learning the answers to old questions, but, more importantly, the increasing ability to ask new questions that may lead to new answers. There is always the danger that old answers will discourage the raising of new and appropriate questions, with the result that error becomes institutionalized, often as a way of life. Each of us need ask himself whether, if our way of life is the answer, may it not be that something is wrong with the kind of questions we are asking? It may be that we will find that we have been asking the wrong questions and therefore receiving the wrong answers. We should be encouraging the retention and growth of that freshness of spirit and outlook that the curious child, exploring the world with wonderment, delightedly exhibits with what often seems like ecstasy. Education as well as educability are in fact socially neotenous processes, and should be recognized for what they are: the nurturing means through which the wealth of humanity is realized in the fulfillment of the unique potentialities of each of its members.

From the standpoint of the student of human evolution, our distinctive educability and behavioral traits are the product of gene mutation, selective pressures, random drift and fixation of genes, hybridization, neoteny—and something more. A narrow biologistic view of human evolution generally stops before reaching the "something more," and considers humans as if they were the products of purely biological forces. Humans are, however, a great deal more than biologized organisms.

The Evolution of Human Mental Capacities

The specific human features of our evolutionary history are indispensable to any understanding of the manner in which our species-specific mental capacities came into being. To ignore that history can only lead to the kind of confusion that many writers on the subject have created both for themselves and their readers. It is important to understand that humans are the product of a unique evolutionary experience, in that they, far more than any other creature has even remotely approached, have escaped from the bondage of the physical and the biological into the complex and ever more challenging social environment. This remarkable development, this movement into the learned part of the environment as their principal mode of adaptation, introduces a third dimension, a new zone of adaptation, which many biologists in considering human evolution have tended to neglect. The most important setting of human evolution has been and continues to be the human social environment, human culture, the learned way of life, the human-made part of the environment. The student of humankind approaching the problems of human evolution must never lose sight of the truth stated more than two thousand years ago by Aristotle: "Man is by nature a political animal."

In the words of mathematical geneticist R. A. Fisher, "For rational systems of evolution, that is, for theories which make at least the most familiar facts intelligible to the reason, we must turn to those that make progressive adaptation the driving force of the process." It is evident that humans, by means of their reasoning abilities, their problem-solving aptitudes, by becoming "political animals," have achieved a mastery of the world's varying environments quite unprecedented in the history of organic evolution. The system of genes that has permitted the development of the specifically human mental capacities has thus become the foundation of and the paramount influence in all subsequent evolution of the human stock. An animal becomes adapted to its environment by evolving certain genetically based physical and behavioral traits; the adaptation of humans consists chiefly in the development of their *inventiveness,* a quality to which their physical heredity predisposes them and which their social heredity provides them with the means of realizing. To the degree to which this is so, humankind is unique. As far as their physical responses to the world are concerned, humans are almost wholly emancipated from dependence upon inherited biological dispositions, uniquely improving upon the latter by the process of learning whatever their social heredity (culture) makes available to them. Humans possess much more efficient means of achieving immediate or long-term adaptation than any other biological species, as we have already mentioned, through learned responses or novel inventions and improvisations.

In general, two types of biological adaptation in evolution can be distinguished. One is genetic specialization and genetically controlled fixity of traits. The second consists in the ability to respond to a given range of environmental situations by evolving traits favorable in these particular situations; this presupposes genetically controlled plasticity of traits. It is known, for example, that the composition of the blood which is most favorable for life at high altitudes is somewhat different from that which suffices at sea level. A species that ranges from sea level to high altitudes may become differentiated into several altitudinal races, each having a fixed blood composition favored by natural selection at the particular altitude at which it lives; or a genetic constitution (genotype) may be selected that permits an individual to respond to changes in atmospheric pressure by definite alterations in the composition of the blood. It is well known that genes determine not the presence or absence of certain traits in the organism, but rather influence the kinds of responses of the organism to its environments. The responses may be more or less rigidly fixed, so that approximately the same traits develop in all environments in which life is possible. On the other hand the responses may differ in different environments. Fixity or plasticity of a trait is therefore genetically controlled.

Whether the evolutionary adaptation in a given line will occur chiefly by way of genetically controlled plasticity of traits will depend on circumstances. In the first place, evolutionary changes are compounded of mutational steps, and consequently the kind of change that takes place is always determined by the composition of the store of mutational variability that happens to be available in the species populations. Secondly, fixity or plasticity of traits is controlled by natural selection. Having a trait fixed by heredity, and hence appearing in the development of an individual regardless of environmental variations, is, in general, of benefit to organisms whose milieu remains static and uniform, except for rare and freakish deviations. Conversely, organisms that inhabit changeable environments are benefited by having their traits plastic and modified by each recurrent configuration of environmental agents in a way most favorable for the survival of the carrier of the trait in question.

Comparative anatomy and embryology show that a fairly general trend in organic evolution seems to be from environmental dependence toward fixation of the basic features of the bodily structure and functions. The appearance of these structural functions in the embryonic development of higher organisms is, in general, more nearly autonomous and independent of the environment than in lower forms. The development becomes "buffered" against environmental and genetic shocks. If, however, the mode of life of a species happens to be such that it is, of necessity, exposed to a wide range of environments, it becomes desirable to vary some structures and functions in accordance with the circumstances that confront an individual or strain at a given time and place. Genetic structures which permit adaptive plasticity of traits become then advantageous for survival and so tend to be fostered by natural selection.

Plasticity, educability, is beyond all other traits the most neotenous.

The social environments that humans have everywhere created for themselves are notable not only for their extreme complexity, but also for the rapid changes to which immediate adjustment is required. Adjustment occurs chiefly in the mental realm and has little or nothing to do with physical traits. In view of the fact that from the very beginning of human evolution the changes in the human environment have been not only rapid but diverse and manifold, genetic fixation of behavioral traits in humans would have been decidedly unfavorable for the survival of the individual as well as the species as a whole. Success of individuals in most societies has depended and continues to depend upon the ability speedily to evolve behavior patterns that fit them to the kaleidoscope of conditions encountered. One is best off submitting to some, resisting others, compromising with some, and escaping from still other situations. Individuals who display a relatively greater fixity of response than their fellows suffer under most forms of human society and tend to fall by the way. Suppleness, plasticity, and—most important of all—ability to profit from experience and education are required. No other species is comparable to the human in its ability to acquire new behavior patterns and discard old ones in consequence of training. To repeat what has already been stated, considered socially as well as biologically, the outstanding capacity of humankind is its educability. The survival value of this capacity has been sufficiently emphasized; the possibility of its development through natural selection is obvious. Natural selection on the human level favors gene complexes that enable their possessors to adjust their behavior to any condition in the light of previous experience. In short, it favors educability.

It should be made clear at this point that the replacement of fixity of behavior by genetically controlled plasticity is not a necessary consequence of all forms of social organization. The quaint attempts to glorify insect societies as examples deserving emulation on the part of humans ignore the fact that the behavior of an individual among social insects is remarkable precisely because of the rigidity of its genetic fixation. The perfection of the organized societies of ants, termites, bees, and other insects is indeed wonderful, and the activities of their members may strike an observer very forcefully by their objective purposefulness. This purposefulness, however, is retained only in environments in which the species normally lives. The ability of an ant to adjust its activities to situations not encountered in the normal habitats of its species is very limited. On the other hand, social organizations on the human level are built on the principle that an individual is able to alter his behavior to fit any situation, whether previously experienced or new.

This difference between human and insect societies is, of course, not surprising. Adaptive plasticity of behavior can develop only on the basis of a rather more complex nervous system than is sufficient for adaptive fixity. The genetic difference between human and insect societies provides a striking example of the two types of evolutionary adaptations—those achieved through genetic plasticity or behavioral traits, and those attained through genetic specialization and fixity of behavior.

The genetically controlled plasticity of traits is, biologically speaking, the most typical and uniquely human characteristic. It is very probable that the survival value of this characteristic in human evolution has been considerable for a long time, by the measure of human historical scales. Just when this characteristic first appeared is, of course, conjectural. Here it is of interest to note that the most marked phylogenetic trend in the evolution of humans has been the special development of the brain, and that the characteristic human plasticity of mental traits appears to be associated with the exceptionally large brain size. The brains of the Lower or Middle Pleistocene fossil humans were, grossly at least, scarcely distinguishable from those of contemporary humans. The brain size of Neandertal man, as we have already noted, was at least as large, if not larger. More important than the evidence derived from brain size is the testimony of cultural development. The toolmaking abilities of Swanscombe man of more than three hundred thousand years ago and the beautifully

fashioned tools of Neandertal man leave no doubt as to the high
order of mental development of these ancestors of ours. However that may be, the possession of a gene system that conditions
educability and the essentially human organization of the mental
capacities rather than behavioral fixity clearly emerged quite
early in the evolution of humans and has remained a common
characteristic of all living humankind. This does not mean that
the evolutionary process has run its course and that natural
selection has introduced no changes in the genetic structure of
the human species since the attainment of human status. Nor is
there any implication that genetic variations in mental equipment
do not exist at our own time level. On the contrary, it seems
likely that with the attainment of human status, that part of
man's genetic system that is related to mental potentialities did
not cease to be labile and subject to change.

This brings us once more face to face with the old problem of
whether significant genetic differences in mental capacities of the
various ethnic groups of humankind exist. The physical and,
even more, the social environments of humans who live in different countries are quite diversified. Therefore, it has often been
argued that natural selection would be expected to differentiate
the human species into local races differing in mental traits. Populations of different countries may differ in skin color, head
shape, and other somatic characters. Why, then, should they be
alike in mental traits?

Answers based on analogies are precarious, especially where
evolutionary patterns are concerned. If ethnic groups differ in
physical traits it does not necessarily follow that they must also
differ in mental ones. Ethnic group differences arise chiefly because of the differential action of natural selection on geograph-
ically separated populations. In the case of humans, however,
physical traits are quite likely to be influenced by selection in
different ways from mental traits.

The survival value of a high development of mental capacities
in humans is obvious. Natural selection seemingly favored such
a development everywhere. In the ordinary course of events, in
almost all societies, those persons are likely to be favored who
show wisdom, maturity of judgment, and the ability to get along
with others—qualities that may assume different forms in different cultures. Those are the qualities of the malleable person,

capable of making rapid adjustments, adaptable, plastic, and supple—not a single trait, but a general condition of flexibility—and this is the condition that appears to have been at a premium in practically all human societies.

In human societies conditions have been neither rigid nor stable enough to permit the selective breeding of genetic types adapted to different statuses or forms of social organization. On the other hand, the outstanding fact about human societies is that they do change and do so more or less rapidly. The rate of change may have been comparatively slow in earlier societies, as the rate of change in present-day nonliterate societies may be, when compared to the rate characterizing civilized societies. In any event, rapid changes in behavior are demanded of the person at all levels of social organization even when the society is at its most stable. Life at any level of social development is a pretty complex business, and it is met and handled most efficiently by those exhibiting the greatest capacity for adaptability, plasticity—the supremely neotenous trait of humans.

It is this very plasticity of mental traits that makes humans unique among the living creatures of nature. It is this plasticity, educability, that freed humans from the constraint of a limited range of biologically predetermined responses. The human became capable of acting in a more or less regulative manner upon the physical environment instead of being largely regulated by it. The process of natural selection in all climes and at all times has favored genetic constitutions that permit greater and greater educability and plasticity of mental traits under the influence of the uniquely social environments to which humans have been continually exposed.

As Hermann J. Muller, Nobel Prizewinner in genetics, pointed out in 1947, "Racial genetic differences . . . may well be insignificant in comparison with the individual ones, owing to the lack of any substantial difference in the manner of selection of most of these characters in the major part of the past history of the various human races." Whether or not we are reasonably justified in assuming that there has been little if any significant change in humankind's mental potentialities during the major part of its past history, it does seem reasonably clear that the effect of natural selection in humans has probably been to render genetic differences in mental traits, as between individuals, and particularly as between ethnic groups or so-called "races," relatively unimportant compared with their behavioral plasticity. Instead of having their responses genetically fixed, as in other animal species, humans belong to a species, *Homo sapiens,* that invents its own responses; and it is out of this unique ability to invent, to improvise, to *respond* rather than to *react,* to *choose,* that the great diversity of human cultures is born. Hence, we would expect to find that the range and average likeness of the inherited capacities of all human populations and ethnic groups everywhere are pretty much of a muchness.

It is by the neoteny of plasticity, of malleability, adaptability, that the made-over ape became *Homo sapiens,* and it is upon the continued development of these same neotenous traits that his further evolution depends. In a Royal Institution lecture, delivered March 6, 1868, "On Some of the Conditions of Mental Development," that extraordinary genius William Kingdon Clifford (1845–1879) pointed out that the first condition of mental development is that the mind should be creative rather than acquisitive, that intellectual food should go to form mental muscle, rather than mental fat. "And," he added, "if we consider that a race, in proportion as it is plastic and capable of change, may be regarded as young and vigorous, while a race which is fixed, persistent in form, unable to change, is as surely effete, worn out, in peril of extinction; we shall see, I think, the immense importance to a nation of checking the growth of conventionalities. It is quite possible for conventional rules of action and conventional habits of thought to get such power that progress is impossible, and the nation only fit to be improved away. In the face of such a danger *it is not right to be proper.*" Hence the dangers of conservatism and the slavish adherence to convention. As Emerson remarked in *The Conduct of Life* (1860), "All conservatives are such from personal defects."

What stands clearly revealed before our eyes in the history of our species is that what has made us an evolutionary success has been our youthfulness and vigor, the willingness to explore, to challenge the orthodoxies with courage and imagination, to affix to the colossal inarticulateness of nature the margin of comment and evaluation that is life's self-criticism—which is mind.

3

Why Are Humans Born So Helpless and Why Do They Remain So Long Immature?

Like a mariner cast ashore
By raging waves, the human infant lies
Naked upon the ground, speechless, in want
Of every help needful for life, when first
Nature by birth-throes from his mother's womb
Thrusts him into the borders of the light,
So that he fills the room with piteous wailing,
As well he may, whose fate in life will be
To pass through such misery.

—LUCRETIUS
De Rerum Natura
54 A.D.

How does it come about that the human infant is born in a state so immature that it takes on average nine months before he can even crawl, and another four to six months before he can walk? A good many years will elapse before the human child will cease to depend upon others for his very survival, a period of immaturity that lasts much longer than that of any other animal. We may feel sure that the helplessness of the newborn infant and his prolonged immaturity and dependency evoked some wonder and reflection among our earliest thinking ancestors. We know nothing of this, of course, before the advent of written history, except for what we can learn from existing nonliterate foodgathering-hunting peoples. In the Western tradition the earliest recorded observation on the helplessness of the human infant is that of the Greek philosopher Anaximander of Miletus (611–547 B.C.). Humans alone, he remarked, require prolonged suckling. Hence, had they been originally as they are now, humankind could never have survived. They must therefore have originated from animals of another, a different, species, that is, creatures who were able to manage for themselves quite early in development. Anaximander thought this different species to be a kind of aquatic "fish-men" who were subsequently transformed into humans. This metamorphosis of "fish-men" into "land-men" represents the earliest recorded theory of slow anatomical transformation. If not a recognition of neoteny it is, at least, the anticipation of an idea that foreshadowed its discovery.

Five hundred years later Roman poet and philosopher Lucretius (c. 99 B.C.–c. 55 B.C.), in his beautiful didactic poem on the nature of things, *De Rerum Natura,* commented on the long-enduring helplessness of the human newborn, as we see from the epigraph at the head of this chapter. He went on further to discuss the consequences of the long childhood of humankind for the development of human society.

> And children easily by their blandishments
> Broke down the haughty temper of their parents.
> Then too neighbors began to join in bonds
> Of friendship, wishing neither to inflict
> Nor suffer violence: and for womankind
> And children they would claim kind treatment, pleading
> With cries and gestures inarticulately
> That all men ought to have pity on the weak.
> And though harmony could not everywhere
> Be established, yet the most part faithfully

> Observed their covenants, or man's whole race
> Thus early would have perished, nor till now
> Could propagation have preserved their kind.

In these lines Lucretius expresses profound truths to which the civilized world seems to have paid progressively less attention. The extent to which the child has played a role in the development of humanity has been severely neglected. The true worth of a people, it has been said, is that seen through the eyes of its children. Awareness of the true nature of the child and of the important role the child is capable of playing in the furtherance of mental health—indeed, the very survival of our species—is, as we shall see, a requisite first step toward the achievement of those desirable ends.

Among nonliterate peoples children are generally greatly valued and cared for, and this must undoubtedly have been true of our prehistoric ancestors. The devaluation and debasement of children seems to be largely peculiar to the cultures of the modern world.

The poet who beyond all others most luminously stated the meaning of the child's prolonged helplessness was Alexander Pope (1688–1744). In the following lines from *An Essay on Man*, Pope expresses in a few words the difference between human and nonhuman infant, and at the same time points to the social consequences of the difference:

> The beast and bird their common charge attend,
> The mothers nurse it, and the sires defend;
> The young dismiss'd to wander earth and air,
> There stops the Instinct, and there end the care;
> The link dissolves, each seeks a fresh embrace,
> Another love succeeds, another race.
> A longer care Man's helpless kind demands;
> That longer care contracts more lasting bands.

Ever since these words were written in 1743/44, virtually everything that has been said on this subject has but confirmed and amplified them. During the latter part of the nineteenth century, for example, the American philosopher and historian John Fiske

(1842–1901), in his widely read book *Outlines of Cosmic Philosophy, Based on the Doctrine of Evolution* (1874), argued that the prolongation of human infancy was a necessary condition for a creature that had to depend for its eventual survival upon learning. Hence, it required a large brain in which to store the necessary information and much less fixity of organization at birth than any other creature. The prolonged helplessness would keep the parents together for longer and longer periods, until "at last the association is so long kept up that the older children are growing mature, while the younger ones still need protection, the family relations begin to become permanent." For the rest Fiske continued much along the lines of Lucretius.

Another writer, who seems to have been the first American to have recognized that the rate of development of the human infant was considerably retarded as compared with other animals, was educator E. H. Russell who, in an introduction to Ella Haskell's book *Child Observations* (1896), wrote:

> It is written that he is "born like the wild ass's colt"; but this overstates the fact in his favour, for the wild ass's colt is greatly his superior at birth. The human infant is, in truth, much more on a par with the lowly marsupials, the kangaroo and opossum, and requires for a longer period even than they the maternal contact, the warmth and shelter of the mother's arms. And not only does man begin life at the very bottom of the ladder, but he "crawls to maturity" at a slower pace by far than any of the animal species. Long before he reaches manhood most of the brute contemporaries and playmates of his infant years will have had their day, and declined into decrepitude or died of old age.

"Crawls to maturity" is especially good for, as we shall see, it could hardly better describe what really happens.

Immaturity and the Gestation Period(s)

Not only is the period of immaturity in humans absolutely longer, it is also proportionately much longer in relation to total life span than that of any other creature. There is no placental mammal that remotely approaches the human in duration of infantile immaturity—not even such animals as the elephant, rhinoceros, camel, and the wild ass, whose fetuses spend a longer time in the womb. The newborn of these animals are able to run with their mothers or the herd shortly after they are born. These animals all have long gestation periods, presumably because animals who are unable to protect their young as efficiently as predatory animals are better protected from external mishap by spending a long time maturing in the womb. As we have already observed in an earlier chapter, such offspring are also better off if they are freed from competition of other wombmates, so that there is a strong tendency for such animals to conceive and bear one offspring at a time. The technical term for this is *monotocous* (Gr. *monos* = one + *tokos* = birth). It has already been mentioned that such offspring stand a better chance of survival if they are born in a fairly mature state. A long gestation period allows for such maturation.

The elephant has a gestation period of about 650 days ($22\frac{1}{2}$ months); the rhinoceros about 500 days ($16\frac{1}{2}$ months); the camel about 350 days ($11\frac{1}{2}$ months); and the African wild ass 322 days (almost 11 months)—each of these is monotocous.

The extraordinary rate of growth of the late human fetal brain, a growth rate that greatly exceeds that of any other organ of the body, produces a head size that, were birth longer delayed, would result in an inability of the head to pass through the four inches of the birth canal. At birth not only are the baby's other organs comparatively lagging in growth, but the structure of the infant's brain is itself in a comparatively undeveloped state.

The great neuroanatomists Cécile and Oskar Vogt and Ramón y Cajal long ago showed that the microscopic structure of the newborn human brain more closely resembles that of the embryo than it does the adult. Myelinization—that is, completion of the fatty sheaths of nerve fibers—is not achieved until the fifteenth postnatal month, nor is completion of the tracts associated with the development of many muscular movements—the pyramidal tracts, for example, which pass from brain to spinal cord. The enzyme systems of the newborn, the digestive system, the immunological system, the body-temperature regulation system, are all markedly deficient. Full development of the immunological system takes about a year; bone development also takes about a year to reach the same degree of development as in the newborn ape. Growth of the lower extremities is delayed after birth for about six months, their growth rate increasing during the seventh and eighth months at about the time when the child attempts to stand. All body proportions remain in their fetal ratios in the newborn, and it is only by the end of the first year that these ratios change and the infant begins to look like a reduced-size adult. By contrast the newborn ape, except for its skull and facial growth, more or less resembles the adult.

No other mammal grows at so slow a tempo as *Homo sapiens* (not counting brain growth). There is none that takes so long to grow up after birth, none with such prolonged developmental periods. When we compare our developmental periods with those of the apes, we find that in every case each period— infancy, childhood, adolescence, maturity, and old age—is considerably more extended in humans than in apes, with the one striking exception being the gestation period. As we have already noted, the duration of pregnancy is, on average, about the same—give or take a few weeks—in the great apes as in humans.

The general tendency in the course of primate evolution toward extension of the gestation period as well as other developmental periods would lead us to expect that, since all other developmental periods are even more extended in humans than in apes, the consequential gestation period would also be considerably extended. But this is not the case. When, in addition, we consider the immature condition in which the human infant is born, it can only be concluded that the human is prematurely born and really should have spent another year or so in the womb. The human infancy and early childhood period lasts twice as long as it does in the great apes, that is, six years as compared with three years; childhood also lasts six years in the human and three years in the ape; adolescence lasts nine years in the human and less than four years in the ape; maturity thirty-five years in the human and twelve years in the ape; and old age about twenty-five years in the human and ten years in the ape. The total life span exceeds that of the ape by about forty years or more. So it should be clear that not only are the extended developmental periods in humans neotenous accommodations to the new adaptive zone of culture, but so is longevity.

The long neotenic infancy of the human compensates in part for the premature birth of the fetus that must be born when it is if it and its mother, as well as its species, are to survive. During the early evolution of humankind, several critical changes appear to have taken place simultaneously. In adaptation to the novel challenges presented by the transition from a forest habitat to the open plains—associated with a tool-making, foodgathering-hunting economy, and the accompanying high premium placed on the development of the erect bipedal gait—the brain grew larger while the pelvic outlet grew less accommodating. The rapidly growing brain resulted in a large head and, as a result of the erect posture, the female pelvis underwent certain changes resulting in a rather prolonged process of parturition. The difficulty arises from the fact that, while the pelvis has widened, the angle formed by the lower vertebral column and the sacrum upon whose promontory the lumbar vertebrae rest has produced a somewhat curved pelvis. This makes it necessary for the head of the fetus to pass between two projecting spines (the ischial spines) situated on opposite sides of the pelvis (Figure 13). The plane formed by these spines and the lower part of the pubic bones (pubic symphysis) is known as the narrow pelvic plane or plane of least dimensions, and it is here that difficulty in childbirth occurs. It is at this plane that the head of the fetus must curve forward through a right angle, and emerge in the axis of the vagina. In contrast to this the fetus of infrahuman primates has an easier passage, since the pelvis is not nearly as curved; the smaller head of the ape, assisted by the relaxation of the soft parts of the pelvis, is able to pass *behind,* rather than between, the ischial spines.

The birth of the baby in humans, unlike in apes, depends considerably more on the three following conditions: 1. the mother's pelvic arrangements; 2. the quality of her uterine contractions; and 3. the molding of the fetal head. During the process of labor, molding of the fetal head is rendered possible by the fact that all the cranial bones remain ununited so that they can be compressed and moved without injury.

The fact that the human infant is born helpless and about one year premature compared with the apes has had the most consequential effects on the evolution of human society, as well as for human morphology. Among the apes it is exclusively the mother

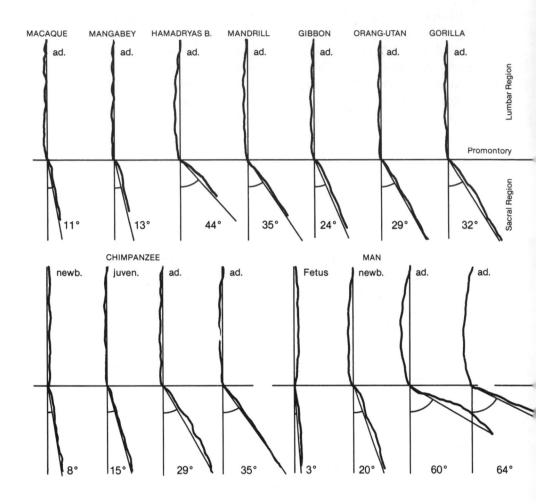

Fig. 13. Evolution of the lumbosacral angle in monkeys, apes, and humans. (After Schultz)

who cares for and provides the food for her infant. In humans periodic sexual heat (the estrus cycle characteristic of other primates) is replaced by the menstrual cycle in the human female, and she becomes continuously sexually receptive, and as Weston La Barre has put it, "the male comes home to stay." The release of the human female from the physiological servitude of estrus, which restricts other primate females to short recurrent periods of sexual activity, made her permanent accessibility to the male the origin of monogamy. The selective advantage of the new family unit on the open savanna is considerable, for the long-extended care of the young is favored by a stable biological-social unit consisting of mother and father, each contributing in her or his own way to the survival and development of the young.

During the rearing of the young there is an overlapping of generations, and the intimate contact between them makes possible the social initiation of the young into their culture.

Cooperation

Professor J. Z. Young, distinguished English biologist, has suggested that with the long, extended period of childhood before puberty, the young would not only be more readily restrainable and teachable by their elders, to the cumulative benefit of the community, but that some of the physical determinants of aggressiveness and noncooperation might well be eliminated from the population altogether by neoteny. These are important points, for nonaggressive, cooperative behavior is characteristic of fetus, infant, and child. In the evolution of humankind there is little doubt that nonaggressive behavior has been at the highest selective premium. Haldane was among the first to point out that insofar as cooperative behavior makes for the survival of one's descendants and relatives, it is a kind of Darwinian fitness, and may be expected to spread as a result of natural selection. As Professor Young has emphasized, the equipment humans have received from their past history is especially designed to ensure communication and cooperation.

That human beings have always been capable of anger, rage, and violent behavior can scarcely be doubted, but such behavior is usually the reaction to specific environmental conditions—not the spontaneous expression of internally generated effects. It is not difficult to understand why, during almost the whole of human evolutionary history, such behaviors have been discouraged. Within the family, the community, and between communities, they would be too socially disruptive. Hence cooperation would be rather more favored than aggression—a fact that is very evident in all foodgathering-hunting societies. Indeed, one would be hard put to it to sustain the view that even in civilized societies anger and rage constitute a "cause" of organized conflict.

In any event, it should be obvious that, whether by neoteny or otherwise, the development of cooperative behavior is the only viable course collective and individual behavior can take. Humankind's capacity for cooperative behavior is seen optimally developed among most of the few gatherer-hunter peoples that remain today, especially among the most primitive—as, for example, the recently discovered Tasaday of the Philippines. Such cooperative behavior constitutes yet another example of neoteny.

Body-Build, Sexual Selection, Dependency, and the Family

Division of labor between the sexes, the female remaining relatively sedentary while the male hunted, probably played a significant role in producing the sexual body differences (sexual dimorphism) that are so marked in the human species as compared with the apes. The relation between body-build and habitual activity and natural selection has been ably discussed by Brues.

As J. H. Crook has pointed out, young women appear attractive to men owing to a combination of paedomorphic features in the female, such as the unbroken voice, the childlike complexion, bodily hairlessness, roundedness of body form, and girlish behavior. This is in keeping with the view, as Crook puts it, "that a greater degree of neoteny has been positively sexually selected in women than in men." What constitutes the selective value of these neotenous traits in the female is that they remain permanently attractive to the male, and thus serve to reinforce the pair bond.

The prolonged period of dependency of the child requires newly evolved social ways of protecting and nourishing it. Instinctive behaviors that protect the young of other animals would be quite inadequate in the human species; therefore there has been evolved in humans what C. H. Waddington called the principle of authority-acceptance. In humans the role of authority-acceptor is brought about by processes that involve the incorporation of that authority.

The long-extended nursing and dependency period would place a high selective premium upon those women who possessed the abilities appropriate to minister to the needs of the child. The bonds that unite the parents and hold them together also afford protection to their helpless progeny, and result in attachment of the young to their family group, thus ensuring their enjoyment of that protection, and the continuing integrity of the biological family. J. Z. Young has suggested that families composed of such slowly developing and behaviorally restrained individuals would be at a selective advantage, and therefore genetic factors involving delay in development would be at a premium. Such family organizations would tend to be the "more efficient in which individuals developed late and were therefore better behaved, in early years because of immaturity, and later by the great development of 'inhibitory' or balancing functions made possible by the growth of the frontal lobes."

And again, as Young has so well put it, paedomorphosis in humans, by producing teachable, cooperative individuals, may well have been the factor that made possible the development of complex societies and their tools:

> By efficient communication man is able to produce a cumulative store of information outside his mortal body and passed on not only to few individuals, as is the genetic store, or that passed by word of mouth, but to many. Each individual thus "inherits" not from two or few parents but from the accumulated memory of a large population. It is perhaps the "multi-parental" inheritance of information that has changed man so rapidly in the past and is likely to do so even faster in the future. Success will clearly be for those populations that are able so to cooperate as to discover and transmit more and more information.

Uterogestation and Exterogestation

It is of more than ordinary interest to note that four scientists— Adolf Portmann, Professor of Zoology at the University of

Basel, John Bostock, Professor of Psychology at the University of Queensland, F. Kovács, Head of the State School of Midwifery, Budapest, and myself—without any knowledge of one another's work (in three cases, at least), arrived at precisely the same conclusion, on much the same grounds, concerning the length of the human gestation period: the idea that the human infant when born has completed only half its gestation, the other half having to be completed outside the womb. Except for an editorial in *Pediatrics* drawing attention to my article, Gould's later discussion of the subject in his book *Ontogeny and Phylogeny* (1977), and a study by R. E. Passingham (1975), the subject has been virtually neglected. Let us, then, proceed to the discussion of this fact and its significance for human development.

Portmann (1944) was the first to suggest that were the human neonate to take the time necessary to attain the state of development of the newborn ape, the total gestation period of the human would be some twenty-one months. Kovács, in a fascinating study entitled "Biological Interpretation of the Nine-Month Duration of Human Pregnancy," written in 1959 and published a year later, showed that in order to be born in a state of development corresponding to that of other primates, humans ought to be born after an intrauterine development of between eighteen and twenty months. Bostock, in 1958, after briefly surveying the evidence for the duration of the gestation period in various mammals, pointed out that two principles govern the length of gestation: the optimum-length principle and the specific-adaptive principle. The optimum length of gestation is dependent upon sufficient maturation of neuromuscular-skeletal development, which permits locomotion and avoidance of possible dangers. The specific-adaptive principle determines that where the safety of the mother or fetus or both necessitates the termination of interior gestation before maturation has occurred, there will be an adequate period of exterior gestation until the stage of effective quadrupedal locomotion is attained. "If," Bostock noted, "the definition of exterior gestation includes the period of maturation from the age of birth to that of effective quadrupedal locomotion, it will in man consist of the first eight to ten months of the first year of life." This usually takes the form of crawling, which the infant generally achieves at about nine to ten months of age, when external gestation can be said to terminate. Crawling depends upon the gradual development of the infant's nervous system, especially the myelinization of the nerve tracts, for function here follows structural development. That being the case, Bostock suggests that the ideal would be a gestation period sufficiently long to ensure optimum development in order to avoid functional hazards for which the fetus is unprepared.

This would at first thought seem to be a desirable ideal, but, as we shall see, there are certain advantages to being born immature. However that may be, Bostock rightly stated that the reason for the termination of the normal gestation period when it occurs is not because it has served its purpose, but because of the size of the fetal head.

Babies require the utmost undisturbed security for a long time. As Bostock says, "Babies must live in an atmosphere very different from that of ordinary everyday living, and its main principles of isolation and security closely resemble gestation itself. It is indeed an exterior gestation."

The evidence provided by the infant itself is no less conclusive. For many months, the infant must be carried everywhere, much as he was in the womb. The major portion of his time is spent in sleep, and it is not until the ninth or tenth month that his sleep begins to approximate the adult pattern. About that time locomotion begins and escape from danger develops. Active contact with the outside world becomes desirable. "Exterior gestation is over: the child can crawl." Bostock goes on quite reasonably to add, "It would seem that every child should have two birthdays—the first to celebrate release from the womb, the second its emergence from exterior gestation into quadrupedal activity."

The periods Bostock has called "internal gestation" and "external gestation" or "neogestation" I have called "uterogestation" and "exterogestation." These terms seem to me clearer and more specific. Uterogestation refers to the period spent in the womb, exterogestation to the period extending from birth to the beginning of crawling or quadrupedal locomotion, at about ten months. The whole gestation period therefore in humans in fact lasts some nineteen months, not merely the nine months spent in the womb. The word gestation is derived from the Latin *gestatare,* meaning "bearing, carrying." The word therefore remains quite appropriate for application to the infant's state of development until he can negotiate his own way from place to place by quadrupedal locomotion or crawling.

Exterogestation, of course, provides a very different environment from that which the infant experienced in the womb; nevertheless the continuing symbiotic relationship between mother and infant in the exterogestative period is designed to endure in an unbroken continuum until the infant's brain weight has more than doubled, his milk teeth have erupted, and he is able to metabolize solid foods and crawl about by himself. Thus, whether we regard this long period of dependency and immaturity as exterogestative or merely as a prolonged period of dependency, it is clear that it constitutes the neotenous prolongation of a fetal state.

It has not been adequately understood how very immature the human newborn is, and how long his immaturity actually lasts. Owing to this failure on the part of civilized peoples, the needs of the human infant during this precarious period of his development have simply not been recognized. Like some larval form that has been deprived of the experiences necessary for its metamorphosis into a mature form, the human infant, deprived of those stimulations necessary for his emotional growth and development, will fail to undergo that transformation into the mature healthy creature he might have been. This is a deprivation we, in civilized societies, visit upon millions of potential human beings, resulting in untold numbers of human tragedies.

For his adequate healthy development the human infant requires, beyond all else, a great deal of tender loving care. Health at a very minimum is the ability to love, to work, to play, and to think soundly. Love is the active process of conferring survival benefits in a creatively enlarging manner upon the other, the communication to the other, by demonstrative acts, of one's profound involvement in his welfare, giving him all the support, sustenance, and stimulation that he requires for the fulfillment of his potentialities for being the kind of human being that you are being to him, that he can depend on you whenever he is in need, that you will never commit the supreme treason of letting him down when he most stands in need of you. It is in this way that one learns to love, simply by being loved, the most powerful of all the developers of one's humane abilities. If, from a purely biological standpoint, we define caring or love as behavior designed to confer survival benefits upon others, then caring, love, may also be regarded as a neotenous trait, for this is what the fetus naturally receives in the womb, and in the human species especially is designed to be reciprocally given all the days of our lives. It may be that religion, kinship systems, social organizations, marriage, and the family, are quite possibly all outgrowths of the neotenous tendency to meet the need for love throughout our lives.

The infant's need for love is critical, and its satisfaction necessary if the infant is to grow and develop as a healthy human being. This need for love—that is to say, not alone the need to be loved but also the need to love others—despite all socially pathological deformative processes, remains the most powerful of the needs of human beings throughout their lives, and it is clearly a neotenous trait.

In the evolution of humanity love has played a highly important role. Except, however, for rare thinkers such as Charles Sanders Peirce and Petr Kropotkin, the roles of love and cooperation in human evolution have been wholly neglected. In an unloving and alienated world wracked by strife and violence, such an idea appeared both unreal and ludicrous. There can, however, be little doubt, especially when one studies the foodgathering-hunting peoples of today and other antiviolent and aviolent peoples, that no early population of human beings could have survived had it not been for the dominant role that love and cooperation played in holding them together. Indeed, it is quite evident that human beings are designed, as a consequence of their long and unique evolutionary history, to grow and develop in cooperation, and that the future development of humanity lies not with increasing conflict but with increasing love, extended to all living creatures everywhere.

It is, in a very real and not in the least paradoxical sense, even more necessary to *love* than it is to *live,* for without love there can be no healthy growth or development, no real life. The neotenous principle for human beings—indeed, the evolutionary imperative—is *to live as if to live and love were one.*

Although it is customary to regard the gestation period as terminated at birth, I suggest that this is quite as erroneous a view as that which regards the life of the individual as beginning at birth. Birth is no more the beginning of life than it is the end of gestation; it is merely the bridge between gestation within the womb and gestation outside the womb. It may be arbitrarily useful to divide up these periods calendrically as we have traditionally done, but it is quite unbiological to do so. It is unbiological because by creating such arbitrary divisions we lose sight of the essential fact that the human infant is in many ways quite as immature at birth as the newborn marsupial, which must find its way into its mother's pouch, there to undergo its exterogestation until it is sufficiently matured. The human infant remains immature much longer than the kangaroo or opossum, but whereas the marsupial infant enjoys the protection of its mother's pouch during its period of immaturity, the human infant is afforded no such natural advantage. This is all the more reason why the parental generation in such a species must clearly understand what the immaturity of its infants really means: namely, that with all the modifications initiated by the birth process, the baby is still continuing its gestation period, passing by means of birth from uterogestation to postnatal exterogestation. The biological unity, the symbiotic relationship, maintained by mother and conceptus throughout pregnancy does not cease at birth but becomes—is naturally designed to become—even more intensive and interoperative after birth than during uterogestation. It is not simply that the infant has a great need of continuing support from his mother after birth, but that the mother has in a complementary manner an equally great need to continue to support and to give succor to the child. Giving birth to her child, the mother's interest in its welfare, in the normal course of events, is deepened and reinforced. Her whole organism has been readied to minister to its needs, to nurse it at her breast.

It is of fundamental importance to understand that exterogestation is not a theory but a reality, for what it means, as we have already stated, is that the human infant at birth and for long afterward is in many ways much more immature than we have customarily supposed, with very special requirements of his own. Among these requirements is the satisfaction of his basic needs. Basic needs, defined as those needs that must be satisfied if the infant is to survive, are set out in Table VI. The infant's organ systems, and his functional and behavioral capacities, have a long way to go before the infant or exterogestate is even partially able to manage for himself.

These are facts we need to understand if we are to minister intelligently and with security to the precariously poised newborn. These are the facts we must understand if we are to help the infant realize its potentialities, and if we are to cease committing the errors we customarily do upon our bewildered children.

While the newborn is in many respects amazingly resilient in the face of all sorts of assaults upon its integrity, it is at the same time developmentally vulnerable and sensitive to the slightest unfavorable changes in its environment. To the baby's developmental immaturity, which renders it so much in need of a special kind of care, may be added the effects upon it of the birth process itself. This has been called *the trauma of birth*.

Whether or not it is true that the fetus experiences its life in the womb as a state of bliss, as psychoanalysts and some others have claimed, such evidence as we have indicates that the birth process is psychically as well as physically shocking to the birthling. Otto Rank, the Viennese psychoanalyst who developed the theory of the trauma of birth, suggested that the satisfactions and security of intrauterine life constitute a blissful state that is rudely destroyed by the experience of birth. That experience, according to the theory, constitutes a great psychic shock, the trauma or injury of birth. Birth thus represents the primal separation and is the cause of primal anxiety. Anxiety is the apprehension of separation. With birth there is initiated a series of violent turbulent changes, not only in environment and modes of functioning, but also a loss of the intrauterine state of security and freedom from effort. The experience is thought to produce feelings of helplessness and anxiety. Theory has it that the severance of the physical and psychical attachment to the warm, nourishing, protecting mother is something that in later life is never accepted at a person's deepest levels. The whole of later life is envisaged as a reaction to extrauterine suffering and loneliness, an attempt to make the world a substitute for the womb.

When the infant has at last come to be born, to rest in his

TABLE VI
The Basic Vital Sequences

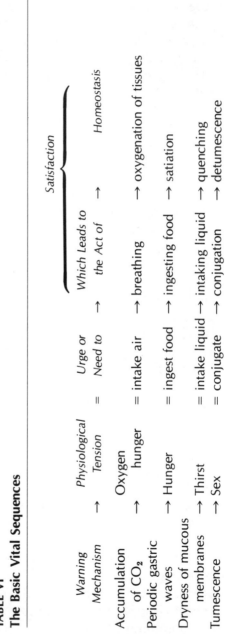

Warning Mechanism		Physiological Tension		Urge or Need to		Which Leads to the Act of		Satisfaction	Homeostasis
Accumulation of CO_2	→	Oxygen hunger	=	intake air	→	breathing	→		oxygenation of tissues
Periodic gastric waves	→	Hunger	=	ingest food	→	ingesting food	→		satiation
Dryness of mucous membranes	→	Thirst	=	intake liquid	→	intaking liquid	→		quenching
Tumescence	→	Sex	=	conjugate	→	conjugation	→		detumescence

Reduced organization	→ Fatigue	= rest	→ resting	→ restoration of muscular and nervous organization
Excess energy	→ Restlessness	= action	→ activity	→ reduction of energy to equilibrium
?	→ Somnolence	= sleep	→ sleeping	→ awaking with restored energy
Tonic disturbance	→ Bladder pressure	= micturate	→ micturition	→ tension removal
Peristalsis	→ Colon pressure	= defecate	→ defecation	→ tension removal
Autonomic activity	→ Fright	= escape	→ escaping from danger	→ relaxation
?	→ Pain	= avoid	→ avoidance	→ return to normal state
Activator	→ Internal Excitation	= Craving	→ Neuromuscular Act	→ Equilibrium

mother's arms or by her side, he looks forward to a continuation of the blissful existence he led in the womb, to a womb with a view, as it were. This is his birthright, for he has spent the whole of his life in close-knit symbiotic relation with his mother, in an environment in which the temperature and the pressure have been constant, and the second law of thermodynamics (which states that within any envelope in which the temperature and the pressure are constant no work is required or done) has been perfectly satisfied. In that environment he lives, it has been said, a Nirvana-like existence. He doesn't even do his own breathing, for that is done for him through the placenta, which serves him as a lung. He lives in an aquatic medium, the amniotic fluid, which is constantly being renewed, and he is embraced by his mother's womb, continually soothed by the regularity of her heartbeat.

It may be that when we speak of a "heartfelt" experience or any of the other numerous "matters of the heart," we are reverberating back to that prolonged experience of our mother's heartbeat during our sojourn in the womb. Research has shown that the fetus is capable of responding to sound as well as to pressure, and that the beating of its own heart at about 140 beats a minute, together with the beating of its mother's heart at a frequency of 70, provides it with a syncopated world of sound. Laved by the amniotic fluid to the symphonic beat of two hearts, the fetus is already in tune with the deepest rhythms of existence. The dance of life has already begun. According to Professors W. S. Condon and W. Ogston of Boston University, as early as twenty minutes after birth the human neonate moves in precise and sustained synchronous organizations of change of movement with the articulated structure of its mother's speech. That precise synchrony with the articulatory pattern of the mother's speech Condon has likened to a beautiful rhythmic dance. A similar synchrony has been observed in children at play, and in adults in various social situations. Condon calls this interaction synchrony "responsive entrainment," and assumes it to arise from processes within the individual. As Condon suggests, the curtailment of synchronized entrainment between mother and infant may, among other things, lead to some degree of learning disability. Although Condon does not mention it, there is some evidence that entrainment in humans begins *in utero,* as shown by the work of Tomatis in France and Truby in the United States.

Theorizing that exposure to the normal heartbeat sound immediately following birth would tend to buffer the trauma of birth by providing the infant with the continuity of a familiar security-giving stimulus, Dr. Lee Salk exposed one group of babies to normal female taped heartbeat sounds at 72 paired beats per minute transmitted through two speaker systems. The sound was presented day and night without interruption through the experimental period of sixteen weeks. It was found that babies exposed to the heartbeat from twenty-four hours of age to the fourth day of life gained forty grams, whereas those who were not exposed to the sounds showed a decrease in weight of twenty grams. There was no significant difference in food intake between the two groups. The heartbeat group cried less, breathed more deeply, and were less frequently placed in the suspect nursery due to respiratory or gastrointestinal difficulty. However, a recent attempt to replicate Salk's findings found no evidence of such pacification. In such matters further independent studies are needed.

Dr. Salk found that mothers predominantly tend to hold their babies on the left side, where their beating hearts sound loudest. He suggests that the soothing effect of the heartbeat is not only comforting but may contribute to the infant's better emotional adjustment in later life. Dr. Salk finds some support for this conjecture in the fact that children with sleeping difficulties, who have required several hours each night to relax and fall asleep, have been enabled to do so within fifteen minutes in the presence of the heartbeat sound. As he points out, sleeping difficulties in children are most often the result of a fear of losing contact with the parents, which to the child means abandonment.

The Technologization of Pregnancy and Childbirth

Contemporary obstetrics, with few exceptions, still treats pregnancy and childbirth as if they were diseases, on the assumption that it is better to treat it as such in order to be prepared for the complications that may develop. Obstetricians have in too many cases failed to understand the needs of the mother, the baby, or the family. An event that should be approached as both a celebration and a ceremony is transformed into a technological medical procedure in which virtually every human need is outraged. Neither pregnancy nor childbirth is a disease, nor should either ever be treated as such. They are—or should be—occasions for rejoicing, events that most of us would regard as such were it not for the anxiety and mystery, the fear of intangible dangers with which our overtechnologized, overtrained, overspecialized obstetricians have surrounded the whole experience of childbirth.

Fortunately long overdue changes are beginning to be made throughout the land. Some hospitals are beginning to convert their obstetrical wings into family birth centers, to which the members of the family can come and stay until mother and baby are ready to leave. Birthing centers are coming into being in which mothers may give birth to their babies under expert supervision and humane conditions. Some obstetricians are beginning to provide similar facilities in wings attached to their offices.

Organizations, journals, and books, all originating from public dissatisfaction with current medical practices, have served to produce some substantive changes. The return to breastfeeding has been mainly due to the efforts of La Leche League, founded by a small group of women in Franklin Park, Chicago, in 1954. There are today, in many parts of the world, similar movements and organizations devoted to the humanization of the experience of pregnancy and childbirth.

Maternal Care

Immaturely born as the neonate is and immaturely developed as he remains for so long a period, nonetheless the newborn human is in every way much more sensitive to the environment about him than has been traditionally understood. "The great big buzzing blooming confusion," which William James, and for many years most psychologists following him, thought to be the limit of the newborn's consciousness and his ability to perceive his environment, is a notion we now know to be quite false. Even though the infant's nervous system is unfinished, all his senses are functionally quite well developed. He can hear, see, taste, smell, feel, and even think, as well as make fine discriminations of various sorts. However, when it comes to helping himself, he is the most helpless of creatures.

It is this very helplessness, so greatly prolonged, that especially evokes in the mother the desire to succor, support, and minister to the infant's needs.

If there is anything at all in humans that resembles an instinct it is the mother's usual response to her infant from the moment he is born. And yet, much as it looks like it, that response is not an instinct, for as we know from many observations on humans and studies on infrahuman primates, maternal behavior must for the most part be learned. Throughout the primates, maternal care is devoted and prolonged. Not only that, it is most touching to observe how among the most tactile of mammals, the primates, the other members of the group respond to the young. Not only females, but males also, will often gather round the mother and infant and beg to be allowed to hold it. This is almost a universal response among humans, except that in some parts of the world there is what amounts to an unspoken tabu on males' displaying anything resembling the interest in children customarily exhibited by women. This is especially the case among the English-speaking peoples of the world, in which the dehumanized and dehumanizing gender role the male is expected to play calls for an abstention from behavior that is considered feminine. The failure here is to understand that such behavior is not feminine but human, and that instead of abjuring such feelings for children, males would greatly benefit themselves and everyone else by developing them. The sex to which one belongs is biologically determined, but what is considered masculine or feminine behavior is for the most part culturally determined. Males do not usually suckle babies, nor will they ever be called upon to do so, but they are able to love and care for babies when they are culturally encouraged or permitted to do so. In many nonliterate cultures this is particularly noticeable. Children in such cultures are seldom out of the arms of some adult or older child. A great deal of cuddling goes on from the earliest days of life, for, since the children have no toys to play with, they play with and care for the younger children as if they were something more than animated toys.

Lorna Marshall writes of the gatherer-hunter Bushmen of Botswana:

> The !Kung* never seem to tire of their babies. They dandle them, kiss them, dance with them, and sing to them. The older children make playthings of the babies. The girls carry them around, not as a task set them by their parents (though they might carry them around for that reason also), but because they play "mother." The boys also carry babies around, give them rides, and drag them on karosses† (a favorite game). If the babies utter a whimper they are carried back to their mothers or nurses. Altogether the babies appear to be serene and contented as well-fed puppies.

Much the same story holds true for other gatherer-hunter peoples. Thus the infant learns a great deal about love not only from adults but also from children.

Children are naturally much intrigued and fascinated by children smaller than themselves, unless, as in civilized societies, they are often caused to perceive them as rivals for the affection of their parents, and especially the mother. In the Anglo-Saxon world, while such situations occur in some families, most children continue to be delighted by these miniatures of themselves with their tiny fingers and toes and wide-eyed smiles. It is only when they reach "the awkward age" when too much seems to be happening to them all at once, that boys seem no longer to know how to relate to babies. In civilized societies boys are not encouraged to show any interest in babies, but girls usually are—hence boys often grow into men who have hardly ever held a child in their arms. When they become fathers and are free to relate to their own children without inhibition, they often behave as if they were making up for lost time. This, surely, indicates a strong drive in the male to respond with caring behavior toward

---

* The exclamation mark indicates the sound of a click.
† *Kaross,* a leather cloak.

the child, even though he may be awkward and far less sensitively understanding than is his wife in doing so. As Lucretius said nearly two thousand years ago, "Children by their blandishments / Break down the haughty temper of their parents."

In the course of evolution a high premium has been placed upon maternal behavioral competence, and so females among the primates, especially because they are monotocous and live in small groups, have by natural selection been beautifully prepared to minister to the child's needs. This has been most supremely the case in the human species, for in no other species is the newborn so much and for so long in need of comfort, support, sustenance, and tender loving care.

Adaptations of the Newborn

In the light of the new knowledge of these matters that has become available in recent years, it is critically necessary that we revise our ideas concerning the needs of both the newborn and the new mother. If we could only realize how profoundly necessary they are to each other, newborn and mother, we would think of them as a reciprocating pair, almost a unity; we would call them by a name that signified that fact—so we shall call them quite simply "the nurturing couple."

At birth the newborn is called upon to make a large number of adjustments to the world into which he is extruded. The placental lung is no longer available to him, and as the air rushes into his formerly inert lungs and inflates them, his respiratory center triggers off the breathing mechanisms, the inflated lungs begin to press against the heart, and in the ensuing competition for space the heart is caused to rotate; the cupolae of the diaphragm begin to rise and fall eccentrically, the duct of the fetal circulatory system between the arch of the aorta and the pulmonary trunk, the ductus arteriosus, begins to undergo closure; the systemic circulation commences to function. The lungs take over the respiratory functions formerly performed by the placenta. The thermoregulatory mechanism must begin to work, the eyes to focus, the sustaining systems to function, and a great deal else.

The amniotic fluid and mucus that have accumulated in the baby's respiratory tract may not have been altogether expressed by the compression of the chest during the child's expulsion through the vagina, so his nose may have to be cleared. The introduction of silver nitrate as an antiseptic into the eyes of the newborn, which is then immediately neutralized with saline solution, often interferes with the ability of the baby to see his mother. In addition, if his mother has received a sedative, anesthetic, or analgesic, the baby may be in a sluggish state, so that even if his mother is fully awake—which she is unlikely to be— they are unable to respond to each other, with a resulting serious loss of communication. Since it is important that the "nurturing couple" nurture each other at this time, a far better practice would be to work for the elimination of gonorrhea, the cause of gonorrheal ophthalmia and blindness, and for the complete elimination of sedatives, anesthetics, and analgesics unless absolutely necessary.

Silver nitrate sometimes fails to prevent the development of infection. When the mother is free of venereal disease there is little need for such treatment, especially in families of good socioeconomic status. When infection of the eyes does develop it is easily and invariably cured by an injection of an antibiotic such as penicillin, tetracycline, or erythromycin.

Reference is made to these details here because it is important for the baby to see his mother from the moment he is born, for there is an imprinting that occurs then that is essential for the bonding, the attachment between mother and newborn, and it should never in any way be hampered. Eye-to-eye contact for both mother and baby is of cardinal importance.

The birth of a baby into a family produces an ambience of sensitivity not only between mother and child but between every member of the family who is permitted to become involved in the event. In establishing that involvement a reciprocity of feeling, of interdependability, comes into being that contributes to their mutual welfare. As Dr. Terry Brazelton has put it, "Eye-to-eye contact serves the purpose of giving a real identity or personification to the baby, as well as getting a rewarding feedback from the mother." A major contribution to the newborn's social development is made through eye-to-eye contact. The eyes have a language of their own of a nature so remarkable, they can communicate messages of a kind more fine-grained than spoken or written language can achieve. As Robson has said,

> The appeal of the mother's eyes to the child (and of his eyes to her) is facilitated by their stimulus richness. In comparison with other areas of the body surface, the eye has a remarkable array of interesting qualities such as the shininess of the globe, the fact that it is mobile while at the same time fixed in space, the contrast between the pupil-iris-cornea configuration, the capacity of the pupil to vary in diameter, and the differing effects of variations in the width of the palpebral fissure [the space between the upper and lower eyelids].

The exchanges that occur between mother and newborn infant consist, of course, of much more than eye-to-eye contact. There are also the communications through touch, pressure, temperature, voice, smiling, laughter, odor, gestures, breastfeeding, and the like.

The Importance of Breastfeeding

In the breastfeeding relationship physiological changes are induced in mother and child that are vitally important for their mutual welfare. Because this is so, every newborn's birthright, namely to be breastfed for at least a year, should become an essential part of his regimen—the regimen of love.

Breastfeeding of the baby as immediately after birth as possible is a phylogenetic trait of all mammals, and thus testifies to the fact that it constitutes a fundamental necessity for the healthy development of both mother and child. That this is indeed so is evidenced by the fact that when newborn animals are removed from their mothers immediately after birth and not allowed to nurse for several hours, the mother is likely to hemorrhage and retain the placenta much longer than when the young are permitted to stay with their mothers and begin suckling immediately. Humans are no exception to this rule. For example, in many cases following childbirth the three problems with which obstetricians find it most difficult to deal are 1. the postpartum hemorrhage; 2. the beginning return of the uterus to normal size; and 3. the completion of the third stage of labor—the detachment and ejection of the placenta. What no obstetrician can in many cases achieve, a baby is usually able to if he is put to suckle at the mother's breast. By suckling, the baby causes messages to be sent to that part of the midbrain known as the hypothalamus, which activates the pituitary gland to secrete, among others, the hormones prolactin and oxytocin. The prolactin deepens and intensifies the maternal behavior of the mother, and assists in the efficient flow of colostrum (the lemony-yellowish fluid which precedes the milk by several days). The oxytocin also assists in this, and in producing contractions of the uterus, constriction of its blood vessels, and compression of the same vessels even further by the contracting uterine musculature. It is in this way that the uterine bleeding is arrested, and the placenta detached and ejected by the contracting uterus.

By suckling at his mother's breast the baby confers survival benefits upon her in a creatively enlarging manner—the definition of love. The baby wants to love his mother. He not only wants to be loved, he also wants to love others. The only way one ever learns to love is by being loved in the reciprocal interchange of love with others in infancy and childhood.

Mother, father, and siblings each grow in their ability to love as they relate lovingly to the infant and child, and in that relatedness they each grow in their mutual love. In this manner is a family built and humanized.

Parental Behavior

We have already defined health as the ability to love, to work, to play, and to think soundly. We have often had descriptions of the unconditional love that infants receive in nonliterate societies from their parents, but though the evidence is abundantly available it is seldom mentioned that children are also a great source of love for other children—not only their siblings, but all children.

Spontaneously the parents, as well as others, begin to behave in a childlike manner toward the infant. The voice takes on a higher pitch; all sorts of cooing and nonsensical sounds are directed toward the baby; faces are made; there are smiles, laughter, gurgles; the infant is cuddled, rocked, and jiggled; and so on. This behavior continues into early childhood, just as some courting birds approach each other with the gestures typical of nestlings, and as other creatures in subdued manner relate to dominant individuals. Natural selection in humans, as in other animals, has so acted as to transform any behavior pattern that is of advantage in communication to another into a conspicuous signal that is mutually understood. In the course of evolution, incidental behavior may become biologically adapted for a signal function. Such adaptive behavior is known as *ritualization*. Among humans the smile is perhaps the best example of a ritualized signal. It serves the function of reassurance, appeasing, or inviting approach. It is socially facilitating. The infant picks up these signals very quickly, and by five weeks is capable of returning a social smile.

As already noted, humans characteristically possess a generalized sensitivity to babyish features, feeling more inclined to care for and cuddle creatures with blunt, stubby body parts or rounded features with relatively large eyes and head. To the neotenous appeal to respond with neotenous behavior even small children will respond to babies with such infantile (neotenous) behavior. As Eibl-Eibesfeldt has pointed out, "The cherishing behavior patterns of parental care have their natural counterpart in the signals that release them, which have been taken over into the repertoire of contact-making and aggression-inhibiting behavior patterns as 'infantile appeals.' In certain situations the adult behaves as if he were a child and . . . such regressive manifestations belong to the normal repertoire of animals. In man it is the same. People who need help or who wish, as in courtship, to elicit affectionate behavior relapse quite involuntarily into the role of a small child." That the child survives within each of us, not as a passing phase but as an enduring aspect of character, is quite as much an evolutionary fact as is our capacity to be kind and tolerant.

What Eibl-Eibesfeldt describes as a "relapse," even though he is careful to point out that he in no sense intends this to mean that such behavior is anything but normal, is clearly behavior that is neotenous, a continuation of behavior characteristic of the child into adult life. As Mary Midgley, English philosopher and critic of sociobiology, has said, "Creatures that have to deal with helpless and demanding young must be capable of genuine kindness and tolerance. This makes it possible for fellow-adults to tap these resources if they behave in a childlike way." Mutual relations, she points out, can be formed in which both parties can on occasion play both roles. "It is at the point," she adds, "long before the emergence of the primates—that nature ceases to be Hobbesian. Friendship becomes possible. And it is on such a foundation (however unsuited to human dignity) that the serious business of social life is actually grounded." The reader will note that these ideas are very similar to those set down by Lucretius some nineteen hundred years ago.

Dependency-Interdependency

The dependency of the child upon the mother and the interdependent relationship that exists between them begin at conception and become a socially intensive relationship from the moment the child is born. The fundamentally social nature of living things has its origin in the physiological relationship between parent and offspring, in the origin of the one from the other. In the mammals the maternal and uterine organisms are for a time bound together in an interactive association, the uterine organism being entirely dependent upon the maternal organism for its sustenance, for the satisfaction of its needs. This process of dependency becomes an actively social one at birth. The dependency of the newborn constitutes a continuation of the dependency of the fetus, a dependency that is critical for the subsequent development of the person.

To be dependent means to rely on some other person or persons for the satisfaction of one's needs. The consciousness of its dependence develops in the infant with the growing awareness that practically all its satisfactions are obtained through the responses made to its basic needs by other persons. The whole of the infant's experience consolidates it in its dependency. The dependency gradually grows into an interdependency, the condition of social being. Growth and development as a human being fundamentally consists in the growth and development of competence in interdependency, in cooperativeness; again, the continuation into later life of a fetal-juvenile condition.

Mother-Child Interaction

As Alfred Adler, the distinguished psychiatrist, pointed out, "The first act of a new-born child—drinking from the mother's breast—is co-operation, and is as pleasant for the mother as for the child." Here, in this act, is the first step in the development of the sense of contact with another person—a pleasure-giving person. Adler continues,

> The child's inclination to co-operation is challenged from the very first day. The immense importance of the mother in this respect can be clearly recognized. She stands on the threshold of the development of social feeling. The biological heritage of social feeling is entrusted to her charge. She can strengthen or hinder contact by the help she gives the child in little things, in bathing him, in providing all that a helpless infant is in need of. Her relations with the child, her knowledge and her aptitude are decisive factors. . . . It may readily be accepted that contact with the mother is of the highest importance for the development of social feeling. . . . *We probably owe to the sense of maternal contact the largest part of human social feeling, and along with it the essential continuance of human civilization.*

New Zealand psychiatrist Bevan Brown has written, "It is obvious that a child's mother is, or should be, the first person in the world with whom he associates. She represents the first *personal* relationship, the first *social* relationship, the first sensuous relationship . . . it would be reasonable to assume that this relationship, being the first, sets the pattern for all subsequent relationships."

Interdependence, dependency, cooperation, social feeling all represent neotenous traits designed to be continued into all the "stages" of the individual's later life, "the pattern for all subsequent relationships." This is both the evolutionary and the biological mandate for all humans and for the whole of humanity. Such a mission takes time, dedication, devotion, and love. The making of a human being is a work of art, extended over many years and accompanied by a great deal of caring. To such caring no creature is more responsive, more malleable, than the child.

Love and Sociality

The subtle alchemy by which love is transmuted in the child into what it most requires for bodily as well as behavioral development may defy complete explanation, but that it constitutes an indispensably necessary communication is beyond question.

Caring for the infant consists primarily in satisfying his needs. Such caring constitutes the commencement of the socialization of the person, preparation for participation in the social group. As the child matures and socialization continues, with its frustrations and bewilderments as well as satisfactions, the child becomes more and more firmly bound to the socializing agents, more and more dependent rather than more free, and this social binding continues throughout life. It is this social bonding of early life that the person is designed to maintain, indeed, to grow and develop in, all the days of his life.

This view of the development of the person cannot be too strongly emphasized. Its implications are of the first order of importance. The conventional view of the socialization of the person as developing toward greater and greater autonomy or individuality is seriously misleading. Of course, every person has a unique personality in the sense that it is never identical to that of any other. Such differences between persons are important and tend to become more distinct with age. This is something to be grateful for. It should, however, be understood that every one of those differences has developed under the influence of specific socializing factors, and that were it not for the creative action of those socializing factors, the functional-structural differences that characterize each person would not exist.

The importance of social interactions, "contacts," of friends, acquaintances, and relations throughout life has recently been dramatically shown by Dr. Lisa M. Berkman of Yale University

School of Medicine. In a nine-year study of seven thousand randomly selected adult residents of Alameda County, California, Dr. Berkman found that persons with the most social contacts were the least likely to die during the study period. When the data were adjusted to take into account age differences, a solid network of friends, relatives, and acquaintances decreased the probability of dying by a factor of 2.3 among the men and 2.8 among the women.

The strong effect of social networks on health and mortality points to the fact that not only do such networks have a beneficial buffer effect on events in a person's life, in addition to the emotional support they can supply, but they also provide the person with important information (such as what jobs are available and how to obtain medical care) and pragmatic care (goods, money, and services). Once more it becomes clear how vitally important interconnectedness is for the health and welfare of the person.

The Myth of the Individual

Every person is socially bound to the group in which he has been socialized. In this sense the "individual" is a myth. Of course, there are discrete objects that for census purposes are called individuals. Such quantitative estimates are perfectly legitimate in their place, but in any evaluation of a human being as a social organism it should be clear that he is as organically bound to others as if he were one of a number of cells comprising a colonial organism. Even physically and physiologically, humans are neither dissociated nor do they carry on a separate existence in any but an arbitrary sense. Even the emotionally arid psychopath is unable to do without others.

In the land of "Rugged American Individualism," in which the focus in the conditioning of the child has been to turn him into a person who conforms to the stereotype of the "successful individual," large numbers of persons are produced who, in the midst of the lonely crowd, live in an isolated glow of narcissism that eventually leads to a chill. The tragic examples of these, in the highest offices of the land, are too numerous and too obvious to mention. There are millions of others like them, and the damage they do underscores the principal danger of the myth of the individual, namely that it neglects to teach the moral obligation of independent thought, the responsibility to challenge unsound ideas and conventions, the right to protest, the bounden duty to object. This is an essential aspect of health. Blind submission to the group has always utterly vitiated personal development and the progress of humanity.

In the concept of "the individual" we have created separateness where separateness does not exist—where, in reality, the genuine condition is relatedness. Certainly individualization in humans exceeds that which any other animal is capable of attaining, but it is an individualization that integratively takes place more fully in relation to the group than in any other living creature. A creature apart from a social group is little more than an organic being. The member of a human social group is a person, a personality developed under the molding influence of social interstimulation. The person is to a large extent a set of social interrelationships. As Bogardus has put it, "As a result of inter-social stimulation he moves up from the biological level. The interstimulation that occurs between him and the members of the group, not as mere individuals but as persons, explains him more than any other method of approach can do." "It makes no sense," writes psychiatrist Harry Stack Sullivan, "to think of ourselves as 'individual,' 'separate,' capable of anything like definitive description in isolation . . . the notion is just beside the point." Both the fallacy of absolute individuals and the excess of individualism, wrote the philosopher Alfred North Whitehead, are vicious. "The individual thing is necessarily in disjunction," he added. And as Gutkind put it, "To think in terms of absolute individuals—absolute individuals are but things—is the outgrowth of our obsession with acquisitive urges. To think in terms of relations is human and paves the way toward the solidarity of mankind."

Distinguished biologist C. M. Child wrote, many years ago,

The individual represents primarily a reaction pattern in a protoplasm of a certain constitution and the kind of individual that develops in a particular case depends not only upon the gradient pattern but upon the constitution of the protoplasm in which it occurs. In one kind of protoplasm, for example, the most active region gives rise to a circle of tentacles and a mouth, in another it develops a head, in still another into a growing tip.

So the kind of person that develops in a particular case depends not only on the gradient pattern of his particular inherent potentialities—that is, his genetic constitution—but also on the constitution of the particular social group, especially his immediate family, in which his development occurs. The responses his socializers cause him to make to the stimuli they offer become the habits that form the unique person. The important point for us to recognize is that the "individual" represents a reaction or response pattern that makes him a *part* of a whole of which he always remains an integral and important constituent. Only disordered persons regard themselves as the whole and the remainder of the world as the part. The person is a product of a field of interactive biological and social forces, and every person constitutes a part of that field all his life.

Making every allowance for genetic influences, each member of society acts as he does because he is the end product of certain historically conditioned forces. Each acts as he does, not because he is an independent individual, but because he is a dependent-interdependent person, bound to his social group by ties that impel him to maintain his relationships according to the requirements, in each case, sanctioned and demanded by the group. This does not mean that the person is without free will. Free will the person most certainly has in the sense of being able to achieve ends and purposes. But it is a will that functions largely within the limits and conditions determined by his own past experience within the culture of his own social group. In the matter of free will it has been remarked that the best *practical* solution of that particular problem is to treat oneself as free and other people as determined. The courteous and honest solution is, of course, quite the opposite.

The "spontaneous" conduct of the person is seldom *de novo*, for however seemingly novel and original it may appear it is usually conduct based on and influenced by models that have been learned in a particular social group. In brief, the person constitutes an interdependent system of social relationships, and it is by abstraction alone that this system may be recognized as a unit.

None of this implies that the group is superior to the person. The obligation of the group, at whatever level, is to the person, to do everything in its power to maximize his potentialities and preserve his integrity as a person, a unique person. The obligation of the person to the group is to contribute toward the development of himself and of other persons. The person is not to be conceived as living for the group, or the group solely for the person; each serves the needs of the other. When this has been said it is necessary to add that this reciprocity is best achieved by the service of the group to the person.

If what has been written above appears as something of a digression, it should be explained that its purpose has been to underscore the importance of the socialization process in the making of the person the child becomes.

The Victimized Child

The long history of endemic error that has pervaded the Western world concerning the nature of the child is only today being very slowly corrected. There are still millions among us who believe that children are naturally depraved, and that it is natural for children to have temper tantrums, that "to spare the rod is to spoil the child." This view of the child, to which many to this day still subscribe, was an article of faith among the Calvinist-Puritan ancestors of contemporary believers. A popular book on the conduct of the household published in 1621, *A Godly Form of Household Government,* put the matter clearly and simply:

> The young child which lieth in the cradle is both wayward and full of affections; and though his body be but small, yet he hath a wrong-doing heart, and is altogether inclined to evil. If this sparkle be suffered to increase, it will rage over and burn down the whole house. For we are changed and become good not by birth but by education.

For a brief period in the eighteenth century, in the Age of Enlightenment, children enjoyed a better press, and the views expressed in Jean Jacques Rousseau's *Émile* had a tremendous influence, which continues to this day. Nevertheless the New Testament view of the child as born in original sin continued to march invincibly on. A widely read children's writer of the "enlightened" nineteenth century, Samuel Spring, wrote in one of his books, "All children have wicked hearts when they are born; and that makes them so wicked when they grow up into life. Even little infants, that appear so innocent and pretty, are God's little enemies at heart."

4

The Child

Although as yet we seem scarcely aware of it intellectually, this contemporary knowledge that childhood is a biologically conditioned phase, of special significance to the formation of character structure and personality, introduces a major shift in concepts and in interpretations of the very meaning of history and time.

—EDITH COBB
The Ecology of Imagination in Childhood
1977

I am not yet born; O fill me
With strength against those who would freeze my
humanity, would dragoon me into a lethal automaton,
would make me a cog in a machine, a thing with
one face, a thing, and against all those
who would dissipate my entirety, would
blow me like thistledown hither and
thither or hither and thither
like water held in the
hands would spill me.
Let them not make me a stone and let them not spill
me.
Otherwise kill me.

—LOUIS MACNEICE
Prayer Before Birth

The thesis of this book is that, as a consequence of the unique evolutionary history of our species, we are designed to fulfill the bountiful promise of the child; to grow and develop as children, rather than into the kind of adults we have been taught to believe we ought to become. By this it is not intended to mean that we are programmed to remain arrested at childhood stages of development, but that we are, by every confirmable measure, designed to continue, throughout our lives, to grow and develop in the traits so conspicuously exhibited by the child.

It should, perhaps, be made clear here that in using the term "designed" there is no intention to imply or suggest a "Designer" or "Great Purpose," but rather a pattern of human potentialities that are polymorphously educable, the result of evolutionary processes, clearly directed toward optimum healthy development.

The child, as a growing concern, pleasurably strives to realize itself. Growth is the principal criterion by which we distinguish the living from the nonliving. But whereas in all other sentient organisms growth is at certain stages of development arrested, humans, with relatively few exceptions within the species, are capable of growth, behavioral and spiritual, to the end of their days. The word "spiritual" is here and throughout this book employed not in any religious sense, but as referring to that combination of qualities that make up the person's attitudes of mind toward himself and to the world about him. This is the secular "spirit" of the person and is unrelated to whether or not he subscribes to any religious system. It is—the need to love others and to be loved; the qualities of curiosity, inquisitiveness, thirst for knowledge; the need to learn; imagination, creativity, openmindedness, experimental-mindedness; the sense of humor, playfulness, joy, the optimism, honesty, resilience, and compassionate intelligence—that constitute the spirit of the child. One sees this spirit in action among many so-called "primitive" peoples, who, interestingly enough, have often been called "children of nature," not infrequently with unconcealed admiration. It is probable that it was the preservation of this neotenous spirit throughout the five million or so years of human evolution that contributed in a major way to the survival of our species. In other words, the spirit of the child is, in the profoundest sense, the spirit of humanity, an adaptive trait of the greatest biological value. It is the omnipotentiality of the child that is so impressive.

It is remarkable how often we speak admiringly of an adult as having "the curiosity of a child," or of "the childlike quality" of a genius or other excelling person, or mention those in whom we simply take delight for "the child in them." I am not speaking of those qualities we visit upon the child and to which we pejoratively refer as "childish," for most of those allegedly childish traits, such as whining, crying, temper tantrums, and the rest, are conditioned in children by the adults whose charges they are. It has been said that humans are the only examples of 150-pound nonlinear servomechanisms that can be wholly reproduced by unskilled labor. In other words, there are many genitors, but few parents. To be a genitor all one needs is to be fertile; to be a parent one must understand the needs of the child and be willing and able to satisfy them. Without such competencies genitors often, only too often, condition their children in the bad habits in which their own genitors conditioned them. It is in this manner that the cycle of "childish" behavior is perpetuated from generation to generation. And because "bad" behavior in children is widespread, what is more "natural" than to suppose that children are naturally depraved creatures? Such a view of the child is by no means restricted to the layperson. In an address delivered in 1922, and reprinted in his book *The Roots of Crime* in 1970, the doyen of English psychoanalysts, Dr. Edward Glover, wrote of the newborn in these engaging terms:

> Expressing these technical discoveries in social terms we can say that the perfectly normal infant is almost completely egocentric, greedy, dirty, violent in temper, destructive in habit, profoundly sexual in purpose, aggrandizing in attitude, devoid of all but the most primitive reality sense, without conscience of moral feeling, whose attitude to society (as represented by the family) is opportunist, inconsiderate, domineering and sadistic. And when we come to consider the criminal type labeled psychopathic it will be apparent that many of these characteristics can under certain circumstances persist into adult life. In fact, judged by adult social standards the normal baby is for all practical purposes a born criminal.

At the close of the lecture in which these profound observations were delivered to the world, Dr. Glover tells us, the lady occupying the chair, Mrs. St. Loe Strachey, a magistrate, protested, " 'But, doctor, the dear babies! How could you say such awful things about them?' " No doubt, in his superior wisdom, Dr. Glover smiled benignly, and held his peace, for he does not tell us whether he made any reply.

I do not know whether there are any psychoanalysts today who would subscribe to such extreme views, but to some degree most people even today hold very unsound views concerning the nature of the newborn. The truth is that by far the most overwhelming weight of the evidence of many years of research by literally thousands of investigators all points to the fact that the child is born with all its drives oriented in the direction of growth and fulfillment in health and harmony. And, once again, by health I mean the ability to love, to work, to play, and to think soundly. It is the frustration of the child's needs by his incompetent socializers that is principally responsible for the behavior attributed to innate depravity.

In nonliterate societies "bad" behavior in children is rare. It has often been remarked by anthropologists who have lived among such peoples that one seldom even hears a baby cry, or observes one sucking its thumb, or indulging in aggressive behavior or other forms of conduct we designate "bad." The reason for this is that children in such societies receive a great deal of love. Babies and small children are seldom out of the arms of others, and even young children delight in playing with smaller children and caring for them, carrying them with them wherever they go. Thumbs do not have to be sucked because the breast is always available, and aggressive behavior fails to establish itself because it is neither provoked not perceived as such, but is treated rather as an occasion for fun; therefore the child receives no training in aggression. Richard Sorenson describes this sort of thing among the Fore, an agricultural people of the highlands of New Guinea.

> There were experimental and aggressive acts by the very young. These were, however, considered a natural consequence of an immaturity which did not yet fully grasp the impact of such actions;

they were regarded as amusing. No attempt was made to chastise or punish; nor was anger or marked displeasure usually shown. Instead the typical reaction of older children and adults who were the subject of aggressive or hostile actions by the young was interested affectionate amusement. If the attack became painful, the subject of it would usually move away or try to divert or distract the young child by affectionate playfulness or by engaging him in other interests. When such "aggression" was directed toward young age-mates, it was discouraged, but, again, not by reproach or punishment but rather by diversionary playful activity or amusement.

The young children's experimental and accidental aggressiveness did not persist; their nascent or aggressive motions failed to find a place in the daily life style. Anger, squabbling, and fighting did not become natural to their lives. Momentary expressions of anger, as might occcur during "accidents" in rough play, were quickly dissipated. Conflict over "things" was typically sidetracked by behavioral habits of cooperative deference or attunement.

For similar accounts relating to aggression in nonliterate peoples the reader may be referred to the book I edited entitled *Learning Non-Aggression* (1978). What the evidence indicates is that there are no fixed action patterns, no "instincts," that determine either the spontaneous appearance of aggression or its triggering by a particular stimulus. This means that whatever genetic potentialities we may have for aggression, early conditioning in cooperative behavior and the discouragement of anything resembling aggressive behavior serve to make an individual, and a society, essentially unaggressive and cooperative. Traditional ideas concerning human nature, especially the doctrine of "original sin," have led us into all sorts of disastrous activities. The doctrine of "original sin" is perhaps the most iniquitous of these ideas. As Professor Herbert J. Muller has written:

When taken literally, the ideas that the whole human race should suffer for the fault of a naïve pair in Eden would seem outrageous if it were attributed to anyone short of a deity. Throughout Christian history the conviction that man's birthright is sin has encouraged an unrealistic acceptance of remediable social evils, or even a callousness about human suffering. It helps to explain the easy acceptance of slavery and serfdom, and a record of religious atrocity unmatched by any other religion.

In the Western world we begin with traditionally inherited preconceptions of what a child is and what it ought to be. The very phrase "raising the child" implies that he is to be elevated from a "lower" to a "higher" plane, so we proceed to discipline what we consider to be its refractory nature by imposing our preconceptions of what we believe it ought to be. From such a blinkered standpoint we fail to perceive what the child is endeavoring to become, namely a deeply involved lover, who is striving toward development of all those marvelous qualities with which he is endowed; to develop not as an adult, but as a child—in other words, to realize the promise of the child. It would be a great step forward if we ceased to regard childhood as a phase of development that terminates at some arbitrary age, and perceive it for what it is, an extended period of growth that slows down, if at all, only after many years. As in all things human, there is a great deal of variability in the time and the rate at which this deceleration occurs; the process of slowing down is very gradual and hardly perceptible, generally beginning in the period around thirty years, give or take a few years.

The Arbitrariness of Our Terms

Terms such as embryo, fetus, baby, infant, child, adolescent, maturity, and old age all reflect quite arbitrary meanings that correspond neither to biological nor to developmental realities. We have already discussed the arbitrary nature of such terms as "infant," "child," and "adolescent." Our terms "adolescence" and "adult" are derived from the Latin *ad,* to, and *olescere,* to grow. But growth does not come in such neat packages, nor does it cease at twenty-one. Indeed, if it did we would all cease to be at that age, for growth is a necessary condition of life. Growth even from the physical viewpoint is not simply a matter of increase in size or weight or amplitude, which at some time during the continuing life of the individual comes to an end. While there is life there is growth. Death is the cessation of growth. It is surely obvious that hair continues to grow through-out one's life, even though some individuals may lose much or most of it. If the cells that comprise our skin did not continue to grow throughout life we would die. The total number of those cells may decrease and undergo a variety of physiological changes, but they are the products of growth and growth con-tinues to the end of our days. This is, of course, true of all organs, including bones. Indeed, if the cells that give form and structure to our bones did not continue to grow we would die, for, among other things, the marrow of our bones is the major source of our red blood cells. The internal table of our skulls thickens, hair grows thickly in men's ears as they grow older, and their eyebrows often grow bushier, and of course there are finger- and toenails. These are a few of the more obvious exam-ples of continuing physical growth into old age. Functionally, at least, one vital organ often improves with age, and that is the kidney. In the mental sphere, tranquility, knowledge, wisdom are frequent benefits of continuing growth with age.

The growth with which we are principally concerned in this book is *human* growth, by which I mean growth of the spirit, the neotenous growth of the characteristic qualities of the child, which appears to be the evolutionary destiny of *Homo sapiens*.

Our arbitrarily fabricated ideas concerning the stages of de-velopmental programming and our conception of them as merely means to the achievement of more consequential ends is unsound and damaging.

As Edith Cobb has written in that luminous book *The Ecology of Imagination in Childhood* (1977), "The dual fallacies of implied permanent maturity and permanent norms, which are now em-bedded in the medical and psychological sciences, cut us off from recognition of the continuity of childhood potential. The fallacies are errors in the use of concepts of time, which subsequently produce errors in ideas of value." Depending, as we do, upon the artificially created norms of growth and development that prevail in the Western world, with strict time limits assigned to each period, we arbitrarily specify the requirements to which each individual must conform for each of these time spans.

This is quite absurd because, among other things, there is a tremendous amount of variability in the rates at which different individuals develop. Here again, the norms of development we have created do not correspond to the realities. We tend to think of "norms," "averages," as if they represented real phenomena, but in fact such a thing as an "average" does not exist—it is a creation of the human imagination, and corresponds to nothing in nature. It is in its variability that the biological riches of a species exist—not in its uniformity or sameness. With our erroneous conceptions of the nature of growth and development, and our typological classifications of the "stages of life," we have destructively departed from the nurturance of human individual differentiation, which, rightly understood and implemented, would lead to a closer approximation of the fulfillment of the highest hopes for humanity than has thus far been attained.

On "Stages" and "Phases" of Development

It is necessary to distinguish between "stages" and "phases" of development. A "stage" is a period, level, or degree in a process of development. A stage is discontinuous. A "phase" is any state, form, or function in any series or cycle of changes that pass imperceptibly into each other in the process of development. A "phase" is continuous. What we have customarily done in the Western world is to arbitrarily set limits to the phases of development and label them "stages." In this way we have failed to perceive two things: 1. that development is always a matter of the context in which it occurs; and 2. that it is a continuous process and not a discontinuous series of periods separated one from the other, each one requiring different kinds of conformities, obligations, statuses, and roles. Such social arrangements are, of course, necessary in every society. It is the rigidity with which they are conceived and the limits with which they are endowed that are false. A genuine understanding of neoteny for the most part renders the idea of "stages" obsolete. As Professor William A. Mason has said, "Because of the retardation of growth rates and the 'loosening' of behavioral organization, developmental stages are less sharply delimited in humans than in other primates. Sensitive periods in development are more difficult to establish, there is less likelihood that the withholding of any specific experience will result in developmental arrest, and there is a much stronger tendency for behavior to reflect a blending or intermingling of different developmental stages, different response patterns, and different motivational systems.''

Certainly there are such things as "stages" of development, for both physical and behavioral differentiation. A newborn and a talking walking infant have clearly reached different stages of development, as have a girl at first menstruation (menarche) and a nubile young woman whose reproductive system has reached full development. Yet while we may recognize the difference between the newborn and the infant who has just begun to walk and (a little later) to talk, we usually fail to recognize the very fundamental difference that exists between the girl at menarche and the woman physiologically capable of reproduction. Indeed, we invariably identify menarche with puberty and the ability to reproduce, thus committing two basic errors in one stroke, not to mention the serious biological, psychological, and social consequences which usually follow from our addiction to outmoded ideas relating to these phases of development. The layperson's ideas concerning puberty are quite wrong, and so are those of a great many authorities, an "authority" being defined as one who *should* know. Every dictionary and encyclopedia errs in defining menarche as the commencement of puberty, whereas the fact is that puberty is a gradual process that commences about two years before the onset of the first menstruation. The onset of puberty is externally announced by the growth of pubic hair and development of the breasts. Menarche is only one manifestation among many of the developing reproductive system, and is not coincident, as is generally believed, with the capacity for conception or the ability to bear viable offspring, any more than the ability to conceive is necessarily a signal of the ability to carry a fetus to term. Quite a number of physiological changes must occur, among them ovulation, before conception can occur, and ovulation does not usually occur, on average, until some three years after menarche. There is, of course, a great deal of variability in this as in all other physiological functions. There are records of girls who have conceived before menarche, although these are rare; some girls are capable of conception immediately following menarche, some at varying intervals later, others not for many years later. Even so, conception is one thing and the ability to bear a child quite another.

What the facts tell us about the reproductive development of the female is that it is a gradual, long-delayed process, and that the optimum period for childbearing is between twenty-one and twenty-seven years, plus or minus two years. It is of the greatest human importance to understand these things because this is the period during which mortality, morbidity, and malformation rates are lowest for infants and mothers, and during which mothers are psychologically best prepared for the bearing of children.

From this discussion it should be apparent that development represents a continuous series of changes toward greater complexity and competence, changes that merge imperceptibly into one another. In development there are relatively few sharply demarcated "stages."

Another damaging consequence of the belief in "stages" is that they are generally erroneously correlated with chronologic age. This practice has become so entrenched that chronological age is not only correlated with developmental "stages" of every sort, but age itself is taken to be a marker of the "stage" of development one is expected to attain at a particular age. "Act your age" is something one hears at all "stages" of development. "Age" is taken to determine "stage," and "stage" to determine how one should act—it specifies the conditions and requirements of behavior, in the event that one should have forgotten one's "age." In this manner, at an early age, the self-fulfilling prophecy comes into being, and one begins to act as one is expected to at the particular stage of development one is supposed to be in, even though one may well feel very unlike what one is expected to be.

At all ages the "age-stage" correlation is damaging, and especially so for children. In the Western world children of the same age are treated as being at the same "stage" of development in all respects whatsoever, for "age" is taken to determine "stage." This is, of course, quite unsound, for every child has its own rates of development, and especially where intellectual development is concerned the variability is very great and very complex. Slow developers have often been made miserable in school because they were not doing the work expected at their age, even though they often later turned out to be much abler than the fast developers. The slow learner may be marching to the beat of a very different kind of drummer. Neoteny may be working rather more to the advantage of the slow developer than the fast developer. The difficulty is that the slow developer in a class of comparatively fast developers may be so damaged by the failure to recognize his individual rate of learning that he may later have great difficulty in making up for his deficiencies, if he has not in the meantime dropped out altogether.

It is a functional error to grade children by age; they should be graded by the measure of their competence to do the work that will be required of them. It should be recognized that a child usually has very different rates of development for aptitudes as well as for learning different subjects and the development of his skills in them. That a child should be expected to do equally well in all subjects at the same time is both unrealistic and destructive.

We stand very much in need of revising our ideas of "the stages of life" from embryo to old age, but most especially of our understanding of the meaning of childhood and its significance for the development of the individual, society, and humanity. The genius of childhood is a common human possession, but it is a genius that is seldom nurtured into adult life except in the most highly creative individuals. These are quite often the "nonconformists," the "eccentrics," who have declined to accept the norms of thought or conduct that their socializers and their society demand of its members. Some, in childhood, are caught in a web of wonder, which they happily never abandon. In whatever fields they later work it is the imagination and the enthusiasm of their childhood that continue to be the source of their interest and creativity.

The autobiographies of creative men and women are often revealing in this connection. Edith Cobb, in her book, presents a list of sixteen pages of such autobiographical works, and in her text illuminatingly discusses many of them. She quotes Isaac Newton's famous account of his own view of his creativity:

"I do not know what I may appear to the world; but to myself I seem to have been only like a boy playing on the seashore, and diverting myself now and then finding a smoother pebble or a prettier shell than ordinary, while the great ocean of truth lay all undiscovered before me.''

The element of ''play'' is a recurrent theme to be found in the recollections of many autobiographers. The description of their work as ''play'' is no mere metaphor, but a genuine statement of what they feel about their work—it is ''interesting,'' ''fun,'' ''challenging,'' ''exciting.'' It is especially this combination of perceptions and attitudes that is characteristic of the child, and, surely, this is not something we are designed to grow out of. Our habit of speaking of ''growing out of'' and ''stages'' of development leads us into the error of thinking that we must leave each ''stage'' behind, placing a barrier between it and the succeeding ''stage.'' This way of thinking obscures the fact that growth is a continuous process, and, what is more important, that we are designed not to ''grow *out* of'' but to continue to grow *in* and *with* most of the traits that characterize us as children. Growth ferments—therein lies its youth. ''The wise man,'' said Chinese philosopher Mencius in the third century B.C., ''retains his childhood habit of mind,'' the kind of observation to be expected of a sage of a culture as old and cultivated as the Chinese. But we in the Western world only too often look upon the child as something of a nuisance, haphazardly thrown together, who has to be subdued into something resembling a ''reasonable'' facsimile of a disciplined human being. And so we proceed to form the child into the kind of person we want him to be. Quite often we are unaware of the fact that this process is to a considerable extent determined not only by what we do, but by what we fail to do. The nonverbal communications the child receives from us are at least as important as the verbal ones.

For example, when a baby is born, failing to realize that he is only half gestated, that he is much in need of comforting after his rather rocky adventure into this atmospheric world, that he is beyond all else in need of tender loving care, we have, in the name of the most ''advanced'' obstetrics and pediatrics, behaved atrociously toward him, as well as to his mother.

The human side of having a baby has not been understood by doctors, although a turn of the tide, initiated mainly by women, is today gaining increasing momentum toward the humanization of childbirth. With the new beginning we can now proceed to the humanization of our understanding of the needs of the child, and in that way, of humanity. As John Fiske wrote in 1883, "We have come to the point we are beginning to see that we may safely depart from unreasoning routine, and, with perfect freedom of thinking in science and religion, with new methods of education that shall train our children to think for themselves while they interrogate Nature with a courage and an insight that shall grow even bolder and keener, we may ere long be able fully to avail ourselves of the fact that we come into the world as little children with undeveloped powers wherein lie latent all the boundless possibilities of a higher and grander Humanity than has yet been seen upon the earth."

A century has passed since those words were written. Today we are in a far better position to implement them than was possible in Fiske's day. Let us, then, proceed to the understanding of the task that lies before us.

5

The Neotenous Traits of the Child

With our additional knowledge of the unused potential
of the child, we are in a position to evaluate the
power of this potential as the evolutionary striving.
. . . Recollection of creative perception and early
learning in childhood can then be recognized as a
remembrance of evolutionary potential, which in
childhood is actually a survival need—the need to
know, learn, and organize. . . . To "become as a
child" is a far more subtle idea than is generally
assumed.

—EDITH COBB
The Ecology of Imagination in Childhood

There is a small boy
in us that we exclude
from the pitiless surfaces
of the mirrors that life
would hold to him.

                Grow

up, is what time says
to us, and externally
we obey it. The brow furrows,

129

the mouth sets, the eyes
that were made for the reflection
of first love have a hole
at the centre through which
we may look down into the abyss
of meaning. But there is that crying
within the young child
who has fallen and will not
pick itself up and is
unconsoled, knowing there
is nobody for it to run to.

—R. S. THOMAS
The Orphan

It is Wordsworth who said "The child is father of the man."
Indeed, as the child is made so the adult will be. It is not entirely
true, but true enough so as to support the common recognition of
the great importance of childhood as the foundational period of
our lives. A modern rephrasing, perhaps nearer the truth, is that
the child is the forerunner of humanity—forerunner in the sense
that the child is the possessor of all those traits that, when healthily developed, lead to a healthy and fulfilled human being, and
thus to a healthy and fulfilled humanity. All the child's needs are
directed toward satisfaction, fulfillment. As we have seen in
Chapter Three, the needs we have customarily recognized, such
as those for oxygen, food, liquid, rest, activity, sleep, bowel and
bladder elimination, and avoidance of dangerous or painful stimuli, are *basic needs,* which must be satisfied if the organism is to
survive. But if the child is to develop as a healthy *human being,*
he requires a great deal more than satisfaction of basic needs.
For the most part the Western world has behaved as if all that he
required in addition to the satisfaction of basic needs were the
disciplines provided by education and religion, or what passes
for them. But there are many other needs or drives with which
the child is born that quickly declare themselves. Because they
appear so early in the life of the child, and many of them are
already present during fetal life, I regard them as neotenous. Let
me set out these neotenous drives of the child, and then briefly
discuss them. The reader is urged to pay particular attention to
them, since most of these needs are not even recognized in
works on child growth and development.

1. The need for love
2. Friendship
3. Sensitivity
4. The need to think soundly
5. The need to know
6. The need to learn
7. The need to work
8. The need to organize
9. Curiosity
10. The sense of wonder
11. Playfulness
12. Imagination
13. Creativity
14. Openmindedness
15. Flexibility
16. Experimental-mindedness
17. Explorativeness
18. Resiliency
19. The sense of humor
20. Joyfulness
21. Laughter and tears
22. Optimism
23. Honesty and trust
24. Compassionate intelligence
25. Dance
26. Song

The Need for Love

The child is born not only with the need to be loved, but with the need to love others. This dual need remains with us to the end of our lives. The only way one learns to love is by being loved. Of all purely human needs, the need for love is the most consequential, for it is the most basic of them. It is *the humanizing need,* the need that beyond all others makes us human. Like the central sun of our planetary system around which the planets revolve in their orbits, so love stands at the center of all our basic needs. The enhancing and creative role of love has never been better described, nor more beautifully, than by George Chapman (1559?–1634), the Elizabethan poet, playwright, and friend of Shakespeare and Ben Jonson. In his play *All Fooles,* acted in 1599, Chapman causes his hero, Valerio, in the very first scene of Act 1, suddenly to break out into the following marvelous panegyric:

> I tell thee Love is Nature's second sun,
> Causing a spring of virtues where he shines;
> And as without the sun, the world's great eye,
> All colours, beauties, both of Art and Nature,
> Are given in vain to men, so without love
> All beauties bred in women are in vain;

All virtues born in men lie buried,
For love informs them as the sun doth colours,
And as the sun reflecting his warm beams
Against the earth, begets all fruits and flowers;
So love, fair shining in the inward man,
Brings forth in him the honourable fruits
Of valour, wit, virtue, and haughty thoughts,
Brave resolution, and divine discourse.
Oh, 'tis the Paradise, the heaven of earth.

No one had ever before, nor has anyone since, so captured the essence of love as these words by George Chapman written more than four hundred years ago.

The baby is born with the ability to love in its own very real fashion, but none of us will ever recognize that fact unless we take the trouble to understand what a baby really is, what its needs are. The baby needs to love his mother quite as much as his mother needs to love him—an interchange in which the father should also happily participate. By being loved the power is released in the infant to love others. This is a critically important lesson that, as human beings, we need to understand and learn: that the cultivation of the growth and development of love in the child should be its natural birthright, the realization that love is a neotenous quality that requires cultivation, support, and nourishment throughout our lives. The essence of love is *giving, caring*. As Edith Cobb has said, "The ascendance out of biological nature into human culture achieved by the individual child is a miracle that cannot be entirely explained as resulting from the power to learn, for it also depends on a child's ability to absorb and eventually to *give* the energy of love." And she correctly goes on to point out that without this step in development the child becomes egocentric, aware of and concerned only with himself—the only world he knows. He never really emerges from his own skin, and remains encapsulated within it, with only faint echoes of the world about him ever reaching his mind. And yet that need for love never leaves him. The hunger remains and, usually being misunderstood, such individuals often seek to fill the void they feel within themselves with such substitutes as power, money, aggression, eating, and the like. In the course of their seeking to fill the void these people often wreak havoc upon others. In the classroom the most difficult behavior problem is usually with the child who has suffered a lacklove infancy. Making a nuisance of himself is his means of drawing attention to himself, in the hope that someone will pay attention to his need for the love for which he hankers.

The unloving among us are those who have been failed in the most essential of all needs, for without love there is no ability to love, and without the ability to love it is possible at most to live a crippled human existence, to remain unfulfilled and unsatisfied as a human being. It is, in short, to suffer the cruelest of all deprivations.

The need for love, at varying levels of integration, represents the evolutionary striving of all living creatures, and is nowhere more intensely developed than in the child. From this central sun all virtues flow, all potentialities are maximized. It is the most perfect of all the conservers of mental and physical health, the highest form of intelligence, and the most effective of disciplines. Out of the learning of love grows the love of learning. In an earlier chapter I dealt with the educability of our species as its most remarkable characteristic, and we need not dwell further on that point here. Love, as Chapman wrote, informs everything as the sun doth colors. It is the prolonged development and exercise of the ability to love that humanizes us, that makes us human.

Friendship

The friendliness and friendship of children is something quite beautiful to behold. Small children are particularly attracted by babies and children of their own age, and will readily accept adults as playmates and friends to whom they can respond as equals. Those who talk down to and patronize them they pass by, but those who respect them for what they are and speak their language, they make their friends. To such adults their responses are immediate. Most adults, however, take the view that children are not their equals. They put them down with age, rank, status, and role; they look down on them because they are small. This ideological view of the inferior status of the child is akin to other forms of belief in inequality, caste, class, race, and similar forms of bigotry. Children are *not* the inferiors of adults, and while differences may afford bigots a convenient peg upon which to hang their prejudices, those differences are, in the child, invitations to others, especially to adults, for understanding and sympathetic feeling, warmth.

While the influence of psychoanalytic theory and the work of Piaget have been most stimulating in drawing attention to parent-child relationships, the richness of children's social relationships has been neglected. These peer relationships are extremely important in the development of the child. Children at quite an early age, three years and younger, are capable of forming deep attachments to other children; these are very similar to the friendships and love relationships of adults. As Professor Zick Rubin has shown in a study of three-year-olds, their relationships are remarkably like the attachments of adult spouses, or the comradeship of adult co-workers, or even relationships between adult mentors and their protégés. Just as adults do, children get different things from different relationships. They provide resources for one another. They learn social skills from one another, and how to deal with conflicts.

The emotional and intellectual satisfactions derived by children from friendships with their peers are critical for the later development of healthy social networks. The friendships young children form are much more sophisticated and intense than has been generally appreciated; Professor Robert L. Selman, of the Harvard Medical School, refers to the tremendous intricacies in their negotiations. Selman has created a theoretical model that describes the manner in which children's understanding of friendships develops in a consistent sequence. From the age of three to fifteen children's perception of friendship progresses from "Momentary Playmateship" to "One-Way Assistance," from "Two-Way Fair-Weather Cooperation" to "Intimate, Mutually Shared Relationships," and, finally, to "Autonomous Interdependent Friendships." The latter Selman describes as complex, overlapping systems that allow for both commitment and the freedom to form other friendships.

It is now well established that children's self-awareness develops by three to four months, but quite clearly babies are able to relate to others even before then; there can be no doubt of the infant's cognitive competence and his ability to enter into multiple relationships. It is a competence that requires encouragement throughout the life of the child.

Friendship is, of course, another word for love, love of varying intensity. The need for friendship, for love, and its maintenance, is never-ending.

Friendship, as a neotenous trait, as love—for without love, friendship is impossible—requires encouragement, cultivation, and the clear recognition of its importance for the development not alone of the individual, but for the practice of good human relations. Parents, particularly, should understand this, and help nourish the friendships of their children.

Sensitivity

How does a newborn baby know the difference between a person who loves it and one who does not? Probably through a combination of conditions. Firstly, almost certainly through the manner in which it is being held, the messages it receives through the skin—its first language of communication through its joint-muscle senses, through eye-to-eye contact, through the sound of the voice, facial expression, and the like. The sensitivity of the child would grow and develop into a most useful ability were it encouraged, so that every baby would grow in its skill in picking up, as it were, the signals it is receiving and correctly interpreting their meaning. Many children retain this skill and continue its development to a high degree into adult life. It is a sensitivity that astonishes those who lack it. They possessed it as babies, but since it was neither recognized nor encouraged it was never developed.

Sensitivity is present as more or less of a remnant in almost everyone; the comment often heard, "My first impression was correct," is a reflection of this. The judgment is generally rendered following a more extended acquaintance with the person in question. First impressions are usually rejected on the ground that they cannot possibly be correct on the basis of so slight an acquaintance, and often enough they are not. The fact, however, that they so frequently do prove to be correct renders the probabilities much in favor of these first judgments being due to something more than chance.

How does the machinery of "first impressions" work? The answer to that question can be something more than conjectural. When one studies over a lifetime, as I have done, the persons who excel in this skill, one finds that they are generally unusually competent at human relations. When one inquires into the history of their childhood experiences it is discovered that whatever the class or socioeconomic environment, and however different and variable their experiences may have been, the one common factor in their childhood experience was the challenge to discover what others were thinking and what they were about to do. Children are constantly being faced with the ambivalent, erratic, and contradictory behavior of adults, of which they have to make some sort of sense and to which they must make the appropriate adjustment. Some develop great skill in deciphering the behavioral hieroglyphics of adults, while others are so bewildered by the kaleidoscopic metamorphoses of behavior confronting them that they abandon the attempt altogether. Some quite early develop the habit of using the individual erratic behavior of others as a whetstone upon which to sharpen their own wits. Others have their antennae constantly extended ready to pick up even the weakest signals, subliminal cues of every kind. All this is quickly assimilated by that extraordinary computer that is the brain, and a "first impression" emerges.

As we have already suggested, the baby does this by putting together the stimulations it receives from a great variety of different sources: touch, pressure, warmth, eye-contact, pitch and tone of voice, odor, manner of feeding, and the like. It is a great complex of perceptions the baby utilizes in arriving at his judgments—remembering that a perception is a sensation that has been endowed with a meaning. It is these meanings, derived in such ways, that form his judgments. It is in the ability to make such judgments that we are all designed to grow.

Women are generally far superior to men in making such rapid judgments; perhaps, as the poet James Stephens said, because they are surrounded by enemies they must be able to see in all directions. Since they have in so many ways been discriminated against they have, compared to men, been especially challenged to develop their sensitivity.

There exist not only sexual but also ethnic differences in sensitivity. In the Western world Jews are remarkably good at this kind of sensitivity, very much for the same reasons that women are. And so are blacks and Asians. What seems "obvious" in much of human behavior to members of these groups generally passes other people by. Hence such sayings as "Market research is a substitute for Jewish intuition," or "Woman's intuition is merely a reflection of man's transparency." Jewish jokes reflect this sensitivity, and psychoanalysis, which has provided the modern world with some of the deepest insights into the workings of "human nature," would have been impossible without the kind of training in subtle thinking that Freud received from his Jewish background. Suffering and discrimination sometimes have a honing effect upon human sensibilities.

Romance-language–speaking peoples are far better at "sensitivity" than Anglo-Saxon–language peoples. Those who have spent their formative years in the lower classes tend to be more sensitive to other people's motives and intentions than are members of the middle and upper classes, and members of the middle classes are similarly better at this than those of the upper classes. The reasons for these differences are entirely cultural. Each of us has eighteen muscles of expression on each side of the face. How we will use those muscles in their highly significant nonverbal ways will be entirely dependent on the complex social conditionings we receive at the hands of our socializers. The face is capable of innumerable different expressions, and the manner of our facial expressions is largely determined by the kinds of responses we have learned to make to the stimuli to which we have been exposed. This is not a passive learning, but an active result of teaching by models whom we learn to imitate as to voice, emotional expression, visual expression, in innumerable motor ways, and in facial expression. It is for these reasons that it is a simple matter for the sensitive person to be able to pick up class differences in infants less than a year old, and in older persons almost with one's eyes closed! The individual who is especially sensitive is also able to recognize the class origins of different people simply on the basis of their facial expression. This is, of course, not always achieved with 100 percent accuracy, but it is often done so well that it seems almost like the working of a computer-like, diagnostic apparatus. To those who are poor at this sort of thing the feat seems clairvoyant, almost supernatural, defying the natural order of things. There is, however, nothing either clairvoyant or supernatural about it. It is a learned ability, and the whole point and purpose of this discussion is to make clear that it is so; moreover, that it is an invaluable skill most of us are socialized out of; to be without it is to suffer an incalculable loss.

The remarkable thing about sensitivity is that once acquired it seems to work almost automatically, literally in a second or two, and, as I have said, it functions with great accuracy. The trait is learned much as we learn to speak. In order to develop the capacity to speak into the ability to speak we must be frequently spoken to; so in order to develop sensitivity one must be encouraged to practice it. Sensitivity is a neotenous trait and thrives on exercise.

Sensitivity is a need that seeks satisfaction in development, and when so developed greatly enhances the appreciation of life. The paedomorphic sensibility of the child is the forerunner of the esthetic sense, of every form of art, of philosophy. Indeed, philosophers have been defined as those who are always asking childlike questions. All reality is relationship and all relationships are enlarged and enriched in proportion to the sensitivity with which they are perceived and lived. Indeed, to be sensitive is to be alive; and the more healthily sensitive one is to the world in which one lives, the more alive one is.

All education should be directed toward the refinement of the individual's sensibilities in relation not alone to one's fellow humans everywhere, but to all things whatsoever. Human beings are the most extraordinary of instruments that can be finely tuned to respond to the greatest variety of stimuli. Just as beauty is produced on a fine musical instrument by a sensitive performer, humans can learn to receive and respond to all those things that cannot be spoken as well as to all those things that can. Such sensitivity deepens the experience of what life has to offer and enlarges our apprehension and appreciation of it.

I have discussed sensitivity at length because it is perhaps the most neglected and least understood or appreciated of the neotenous traits with which the newborn is endowed.

The Need to Think Soundly

Strangely enough, it is not generally understood that the ability to think soundly is almost as vitally necessary as the ability to breathe soundly. There are untold numbers of individuals who do not breathe normally, who are shallow breathers, much to the detriment of their health. Nevertheless they survive, even though they suffer from various deficits as a consequence. Unsound thinking leads to unsound conduct; unsound conduct adversely affects health, especially mental health, and results in human as well as socially destructive effects. Thinking soundly leads to the understanding of the necessity of feeling soundly. In the greater part of the civilized world men have long been bent on a course of self-destruction largely as a consequence of the trained inability to think soundly.

The brain, as we have already seen, is a problem-solving organ; as such it requires constant exercise. That exercise is largely of a problem-solving kind. Thinking when reduced to its elements is principally a problem-solving process. Problems are solved by sound thinking. Unsound thinking leads to unsound "solutions," and a mind constructed of such unsound "solutions" to fundamental human problems is not likely to do itself or anyone else any good—and by "good" here I mean the ability to produce or contribute to a healthy human environment. It is thinking that makes the greatness of man, said Pascal, but too many of us really do not think; what so many of us do, without being aware of the fact, is to employ words, stereotypes, clichés, prejudices, as substitutes for thinking. As Jane Taylor (1783–1827), English poet and author, wrote:

> Though man a thinking being is defined,
>   Few use the grand prerogative of mind,
> How few think justly of the thinking few!
>   How many never think, who think they do!

Too much of our learning is done without thought, and such learning is labor lost. Our schools are severely to blame here, for there is little or no education in them. What passes for education is largely instruction, training in the skills and techniques of the three "R's." Too often "education" consists in teaching children *what* to think, rather than *how* to think. We don't give children problems to solve. We give them answers to remember. We cause them to engorge quantities of rote-memorized facts, and then to disgorge them on certain ritual occasions onto blank sheets of paper (thus leaving their minds more or less blank forever thereafter). Those who have the highest disgorgative abilities are considered the brightest and the best, and are the most highly rewarded. This kind of "education" in fact represents one of the last surviving forms of ritual slaughter, tending to undermine the ability to think. As one proceeds from Bachelor's degree to Master's and Doctor's degrees, one dies both intellectually and spiritually by degrees.

Rote-rememberers are seldom capable of thinking except in limited sorts of ways on intermittent occasions, and they are seldom capable of reading, for they read, if they read at all, largely with the eye, and rarely with the mind. Reading tends to be indulged in as an anodyne rather than as a pleasurable stimulus to the mind and the enlargement of experience, for the mind grows by what it feeds on. The initiation of the habit of reading early in the life of the child can be made an exciting experience, which should, of course, be a pleasurable one for the parents as well as for the child. It can be among the most delightful, sharing, and enhancing of encounters. It should, therefore, never be approached as a chore or a duty, for perfunctoriness does not greatly recommend itself to the child. Children who are read to as a duty will receive an uninviting impression of the purpose of reading. Children enjoy nothing more than being read to, when the reader enjoys the reading and communicates his enthusiasm to the child. "Tell me a story" is the universal appeal of the child, and is, of course, the principal reason for the enduring popularity of children's books. Such books as Lewis Carroll's *Alice in Wonderland,* Kenneth Graham's *The Wind in the Willows,* Antoine Saint-Exupéry's *The Little Prince,* E. B. White's *Charlotte's Web,* Munro Leaf's *Ferdinand the Bull,* though written for children, enjoy their greatest readership among adults. And the reason for this is not far to seek: it is the nostalgic delight that we take in the recovery of the world of childhood, the wonderland, the land of dreams, the recreation of myth.

> Go, said the bird, for the leaves
>   were full of children,
> Hidden excitedly, containing laughter,
>   Go, go go, said the bird: humankind
> Cannot bear very much reality.
>
> T. S. ELIOT *Burnt Norton*

In passing it is worth noting that most of these books depend for their success on children's love of animals—a neotenous trait.

The reading of stories to children is not only an important educational experience for the child, but also an opportunity for firmer bonding between parent and child: an opportunity to answer all sorts of questions that come to the child's mind, and to raise new ones. The shared experience in storytelling, of reading as it were together, constitutes the best introduction to reading even before the child can spell. Being read to will make him all the more ready and anxious to read for himself; and if he has been read to in an interested and interesting manner, his mind will become all the more quickly the sensitive information-processing and -analyzing system it is capable of being. Assimilating what he hears, he responds increasingly more appropriately to new and enlargingly more complex inputs.

Children love to think. They hunger to do so. Indeed, the whole course of the child's life is an unending process of problem-solving. And this commences almost from the moment the child is born. It is exciting to watch the development of the first manifestations of thought during the first hours of life, the intense visual pursuit of objects moving across the newborn's visual field, the scanning of contours and geometrical figures, as well as the studied scrutiny of the mother's face.

One should always remember that while the urge to think is a powerful drive in the child, he must *learn* to think, and therefore the child requires the necessary encouragement to think, and to think soundly: to be taught early in life that there are few if any absolute truths, but mainly more or less high degrees of probability, which one constantly tries to improve; that the method of sound thinking is not simply *verification,* but more importantly, *falsification.* Falsification is the highly critical examination of all received "truths" and of new theories by looking for what, if anything, would show them to be false. It is only when such "truths" and theories are able to withstand our critical treatment that we can ever be reasonably sure that their claims are worth taking seriously. The difference between those who think soundly and those who accept things on faith is that thinkers, like scientists, believe in proof without certainty, while those who put their trust in faith believe in certainty without proof. The child is equipped with all the potentialities for sound thinking: his curiosity, wonder, explorativeness, experimental-mindedness, openmindedness, and so on, all are ready for the exercise they require. In an age of technology it is often forgotten that the most powerful of power tools is the human brain.

With the advent of TV, too many of us are watching life instead of living it. Hence it is more than ever necessary to understand that this "chewing-gum of the mind," this "lobotomy-box," at which children are spending more hours than they spend at school, which is robbing them of their childhood, must not be allowed to serve as a substitute for the homework they should be doing. Nor must it be allowed to prevent the exercise of the muscles of the mind as well as those of the body, for both kinds of exercise are (or should be) sports.

It was Socrates who said that the unexamined life is not worth living, and, indeed, no one can call himself a truly civilized human being who does not from time to time examine his first principles. All good observation is analytic and experimental, and all thought should be a constant testing and checking. This kind of busy thinking is one of the great delights of life, and nothing is calculated to keep one more young-minded than the energetic and lively exercise of hard thinking. The harder one works at such thinking, the more pleasurable, the more exhilarating, the more rewarding it is. That is why so many of the world's greatest thinkers are like children about their work—greedy for more, just as the neotenous child is.

The Need to Know

The need to know is not the same as the need to learn. To know is to have a clear perception or understanding. To learn is to fix in the mind. The two, in any person, may or may not be related. It is possible to learn without knowing. But in the child the two do go together. The child wants to know and to learn to know, as well as to know how to learn. A few hours or so after he is born the human infant declares his need to know. The manner in which he establishes eye-contact with his mother, the way in which he scans her face is evidence of his interest in absorbing the information he needs for both immediate and future use. He is establishing the compass points, as it were, that will enable him to recognize and distinguish the objects of his experience. Learning is, of course, involved in this, but the drive is to know. The need to know is a first-order evolutionary drive—vital for survival and development. What the infant is doing in knowing is endowing sensations with meaning; that is, converting raw sensations into perceptions. In short, he is engaged in an active process of organization, of understanding, of becoming aware. It is by this kind of "knowing" that the child "becomes." In contact with his mother's body at the breast, he absorbs a great variety of information. Tennyson resumed it beautifully in his poem *In Memoriam* (published in 1850, but written a good deal earlier):

> The baby new to earth and sky
> What time his tender palm is prest
> Against the circle of the breast,
> Has never thought that "this is I."

> But as he grows he gathers much,
> And learns the use of "I" and "me,"
> And finds "I am not what I see,
> And other than the things I touch."

> So rounds he to a separate mind
> From whence clear memory may begin,

And thro' the frame that binds him in
His isolation grows defined.

This use may lie in blood and breath,
Which else were fruitless of their due,
Had man to learn himself anew
Beyond the second birth of Death.

In this manner, by discriminating the other half of himself, the infant becomes himself. But the distinction is not the individuation of separation, but rather of *identification,* often of losing oneself within the object that one knows very well has a unique and independent existence. One comes to rejoice in that uniqueness as an enrichment both for the other and of oneself.

It is the development of this double process that enables us in all later periods of our lives to identify ourselves, to lose ourselves, to become for a time whatever we may admire—a landscape, a painting, a poem, the picturesque, music, someone we love, a friend, whatever. To know is to be—"I think, therefore I am"—and to become and (what is extremely important to understand) to be involved. And what is talent, if not to a large extent involvement? It is deep involvement that characterizes the need to know and the exercise of that need.

As individuals and as a species we are clearly designed to acquire a great deal of knowledge, and not to remain in that voluntary state of blinkered ignorance that characterizes so many who enjoy all the opportunities in the world to enlarge their minds and increase their knowledge. Most ignorance is voluntary, and there is no health in that, only narrowness, impoverishment of spirit, and bigotry. Such persons resemble the pupil of the human eye; the more light you expose them to, the narrower they grow. It is a disastrous self-limitation, at all costs to be prevented.

The world is so full of wonderful things we should all, if we were taught how to appreciate it, be far richer than kings. The conventional means, however, by which we are instructed in the acquisition of "knowledge" both in the home and in school generally constitute the greatest impediment to the acquisition of a love of knowledge. School, instead of being a magic casement that opens on unending vistas of excitement, has become a restrictive, linear, one-dimensional, only too often narrowing experience, and to many a dead loss; hence the large number of dropouts. They drop out because they do not find enough to interest them in school; they find little or nothing that is relevant to their lives, that will prepare them for life; in short, because they are bored they drop out.

Dull teachers and threadbare curricula are not for lively minds. If school, if education, cannot be made excitingly interesting by any teacher, then that teacher should realize that he or she is in the wrong profession, for the child has not yet been born who cannot be interested in the adventure of knowing, the excitement of ideas.

There is great pleasure in the acquisition of knowledge, even expertise, for its own sake, even as an end in itself; but to experience such pleasure one must be genuinely interested. Our object should always be to put the best that we have in the service of the best that we know. What we know about anything is the way we behave about it. People collect all sorts of things upon which they often become experts; some collect ideas and become intellectuals, others go fishing and end up presenting magnificent collections of everything relating to piscatorial enchantments to libraries, and so on. To increase one's knowledge in these ways is to enlarge one's mind and energize one's spirit.

The Need to Learn

What is the need to learn? It is essentially the need to become aware, to increase the dimensions of one's consciousness, to increase in the strength of any act through repetition. One has to learn to behave as a human being. One has to learn to learn, even though the urge to learn, the need to learn, is there from the moment of birth, if not before. We know that the fetus is already capable of learning in the womb, and that learning, continued throughout life, is the principal means by which we develop our faculties and become functioning social human beings. The child is the most avid learner of all living things on this earth. Learning requires not only information processing and analyzing, but also ordering and classification. The process is one of discovery, the perception of patterns in relations, and the distinction between those that work and those that don't. In later life this is precisely what the scientific mind does and the artist accomplishes. Learning in this sense is essentially a creative process; unfortunately that is not as modern "education" sees it. Contemporary "education," teaching with its emphasis on rote learning, takes the essential element, the creativity, out of learning and renders it mere instruction in technical skills. Primarily, learning should be not for the purpose of accumulating facts, techniques, and skills, but for the living of life. In the Western world we make too much of a business of learning, instead of seeing it as a way to a fuller life, with the result that we end up by making business a way of life instead of a way of earning a living. All learning is continual development and adaptation inextricably bound together, a very strong neotenous bond, without which there would be no genuine life, merely existence. Even existence would be impossible without learning, for every living thing has to learn to adapt itself to its environment, and humans more so than any other creature, for everything we come to do *as* human beings—that is, those things that no other creature is capable of doing—we have to learn from other human beings. Above all, as I have already said, we have to learn to be human. That is, of course, the greatest and most important of all the arts and all the skills.

All this we should have learned by the time we reach adolescence, if not long before. Learning to live may turn into a passion to learn. That is something to cultivate quite early in life. Such passion, as the realization of a neotenous drive, enriches life and keeps the mind interested, involved, lively, and young. As the mind is pitched the spirit is pleased.

If one has failed to acquire an enthusiasm for learning, it is never too late to begin. But first one must be interested in beginning. This means finding something in which to be interested, and then cultivating it as one would cultivate one's garden. Something to work at with the promise of a good harvest; something mind-challenging, requiring application and some commitment. An example would be reading in some subject, which should, in any event, always be the foundation of informed opinion and action. Not that well-chosen TV programs cannot be of the greatest help. There are many such programs, and there are even such things as sunrise seminars, which are usually well organized and well delivered. These should not be underestimated. It is well worth taking the trouble to find these programs, as well as others that can be helpful and stimulating. Wherever possible, discussion groups should be organized on a frequent and regular basis. And, of course, attending intellectually stimulating lectures is a great help. Good movies, good theater, the ballet, dance, art galleries and museums, good periodicals of every sort, all substantially contribute to that human literacy that is at once the most vital and the most rejuvenating of all our accomplishments. We learn by looking toward the future, and how we learn and what we learn will to a great extent influence that future. "Life," E. M. Forster wrote, "is a public performance on the violin, in which you must learn the instrument as you go along." It need not be so. Always remember Goethe's words: "One never learns to understand truly anything but what one loves." The child who learns to love will love to learn.

The Need to Work

"Men," observed Dryden, "are children of a larger growth." True, but growth as a human being is a very gradual process. It is not self-propelled, but requires a great deal of work—work that begins at birth, and, if one is to continue to grow, is neverending. Growing is a work of art, an art in which one grows with the quality and dedication of the work one puts into it. As a work of art the work of growing has an esthetic aspect, which is—or should constitute—an intrinsic part of it, a skill, an efficiency, and a beauty, all of which contribute to the joy of healthy living.

Even before he is born the work of living begins for the baby, when, during the process of labor, he is besieged with more sensory stimuli than it would seem possible to manage and respond to in motor acts. While clearly at the mercy of physiological processes designed to expel him from the womb, the baby is challenged to work at contriving to survive the adventure. If he doesn't work, he won't survive. Most babies do the necessary work and survive. From birth onward the baby is clearly *striving* to survive. This entails a great deal of activity, a considerable amount of work on his part. From the crying to the breathing he must do for the first time, to the surveying of the brave new world in which he has now become a participating member, to the suckling, and so on, all this, and more, entails work— meaning by "work" physical or mental effort in order to do something. The baby is soon confirmed in his drive that work can be pleasurable, and what more pleasurable work can there be than to lie in one's mother's arms suckling at her breast, absorbing her nourishment and warmth, and exchanging all those pleasant communications that go on between mother and infant? It is a pleasure that is renewed in other forms of work throughout one's life. But whether one has been breastfed or not, work is a pleasure that is never lost.

Children love to work from the earliest ages on, and should be trained early in the habit of work—not merely for its own sake, but for the sake of getting done things that must be done in order to grow in the competence of a healthy human being. Work graduated to the capacities of the child should be a regular part of his life, so that he becomes disciplined in the art of work as a pleasure rather than as a chore or an affliction.

The perception of work as pleasure, freedom, and responsibility is the natural development of the disciplined human being. And by discipline I mean the training that develops self-control, character, orderliness, and efficiency, the discipline that matters most—not that which is imposed from without, but that which emanates from within. It is through the habit of work that the disciplined development of all our traits may be most effectively achieved.

To neglect the cultivation and growth of the habit of work in the child is to deprive him of one of the most important neotenous traits, without which healthy growth and development are impossible. It was the French poet Charles Baudelaire (1821– 1867) who remarked, "How many years of fatigue and punishment it takes to learn the simple truth that work, that disagreeable thing, is the only way of not suffering in life, or at all events of suffering less." As Aldous Huxley (1894–1963) said, "Creative work, of however humble a kind, is the source of man's most solid, least transitory happiness." And Chekhov (1860– 1904): "Work, my dear, is the only thing we really have, apart from one another." Also John Stuart Mill (1806–1873) wrote, "Ask your self whether you are happy, and you cease to be so. The only chance is to treat, not happiness, but some end external to it, as the purpose of life. Let your self-consciousness, your scrutiny, your self-interrogation exhaust themselves on that; and if otherwise fortunately circumstanced you will inhale happiness with the air you breathe, without dwelling upon it or thinking about it, or putting it to flight by fatal questioning." And, of course, if you set out to seek happiness it is not very likely you will find it, for happiness usually comes by the way as a product of something, usually work, well done. Work brings its own relief. It is also the surest defense against boredom and drudgery. Blessed, indeed, are those who have found their work, for they shall inherit the only kingdom of heaven that is to be found this side of paradise.

The ability to work is, of course, one of the necessary conditions of mental health. Among our most important tasks in child-rearing should be the early teaching of habits of work. Yet this is one of the most neglected aspects of child-rearing in America, and has been for so many years in the land in which there has been a mass desertion of the agrarian way of life for that of the city. In agrarian America children were, from sheer necessity, taught the virtues of hard work. Today the emphasis has shifted largely to "getting by" with as little work as possible. Homework is regarded as a drag, and is performed in an uninvolved, perfunctory manner; school is felt to be an unavoidable, burdensome thing. Parents want to make life easy for their children, without understanding that by doing so they are in fact making it difficult for them. Parents need to understand that when children are early encouraged in their need to work, they find work pleasurable and rewarding. Until parents learn this, and the whole of our miscalled "educational system" is revised toward making work, among other things, a pleasurable experience, we shall continue to fail our workers in developing one of the most valuable of their potential abilities—creativity.

The habit of work can become a pleasure to which one looks forward with eagerness. Founded early in life, this habit makes easier everything one does later in life. What is work? It is purposeful activity, mental or physical effort designed to do or make something. Work may often involve burdensome and troubling effort, but when sensibly taught the child can come to see that the burden and the trouble together constitute a genuine part of the pleasure one takes in satisfactorily completing a task. What, indeed, would life be without effort, without work? Very empty indeed, as are the lives of many who don't have to work for a living. Nothing more destructive can befall a man than to be deprived of employment. An old German proverb says that work makes life sweet. It does that, indeed, but it does a great deal more: it gives life a great part of its meaning. Not work in its narrow sense, but work conceived as a continuing adventure of ever-new challenges in problem-solving.

There is work that some people find boring or monotonous—I imagine it would be difficult to find the assembly line other than that. But even the challenges presented by the assembly line are probably frequent enough to require some mental effort. Those who are employed in tedious or boring work soon begin to find it wearisome and ungratifying—the very opposite of what work should be. The trick is to make the work, however intrinsically dull or vapid, as interesting as an interested mind can make almost anything, and that is an ability that can be taught and learned.

Interest is the road to understanding, for in order to understand anything one must be interested. The child's interest knows no boundaries. It is the disciplined cultivation of that interest that is the best insurance against boredom of any kind in every connection, even against bores, for the ability to think soundly can be depended upon to provide solutions even to such dire contingencies. To be interested is not only pleasant and enhancing but also to be interesting, and while we have here been discussing how the child should be encouraged to grow in his interests because they are so fulfilling, what can we say for those of older years who have been failed in their need to think soundly, who have been raised on a fake substitute, and who desire to rethink themselves?

The Need to Organize

Very shortly after birth it is quite clear that the newborn is attempting to organize what he is experiencing. He scans his mother's face, he fixes on her eyes, follows her movements, and synchronizes his own with them; he imitates and responds very quickly to a variety of stimuli—all of which take some organizing. The organizing trait expresses itself in more extended form quite early in childhood in the form of the collection, arrangement, and classification of various objects, and in the strong tendency to put things in their proper order. It is a trait that is often mistaken for "tidiness," when in fact it is quite another thing. The possessor of a well-organized mind may be quite untidy in his personal habits. The untidy laboratory or desk of the distinguished scientist is a well-known example of the non-correlation between mental organization and tidiness—not that the two are incompatible. Indeed, they often go together, but as I have said, they are not the same things. As T. H. Huxley remarked, science is nothing but trained and organized common sense—which, it may be added, has no necessary connection with the state of the scientist's desk, but only with his mind.

I have even heard one distinguished scientist, whose whole study looked as if several hurricanes as well as a couple of tornadoes had hit it, say that a tidy desk was a sign of an untidy mind! I believe that he was at least half-serious. While it seemed that the mountain of letters, manuscripts, notes, periodicals, and other impedimenta would have made it impossible to find anything, he was nonetheless able to lay hands on whatever he wanted. But perhaps there was some sort of organization to the unconformable geological strata of what seemed to others like utter chaos. In any event, it is not the child's way of doing things. Children tend to be naturally tidy-minded and neatly order the things about them. Yet this is another trait that is little recognized, and for the most part tends to receive little encouragement. Parents, and especially mothers, are continually urging their children to be tidy, and often enough set them good examples. In the Western world boys tend to be untidy, while girls tend to be conspicuously more orderly than boys. Tidiness is a great virtue, and should, of course, be cultivated, but as I have said, it should not be confused with organization, even though it is a species of organization. The organization of one's ideas, the systematizing of one's thought, and the consistency with which one holds one's views on various matters should be subject to re-examination, without falling victim to that hobgoblin of little minds, as Emerson put it: a foolish consistency. Too much of a good thing is never any good, and even the wise through an excess of wisdom are made foolish; so, nothing in excess.

Habits of organization and tidiness in all respects whatever are essential both to the well-ordered life and the well-organized mind, always remembering, however, that the natural rhythm of human life is not a slavish routinism but the enjoyment of variety. As Montaigne put it, "There is no course of life so weak and sottish as that which is managed, by order, method, and discipline." Children know how to vary their enjoyments, a trait that is often mistaken by their elders as inconstancy, lack of concentration, unseriousness, and the like.

> Order is a lovely thing;
> On disarray it lays its wing,
> Teaching simplicity to sing.
> ANNA HEMPSTEAD BRANCH
> *The Monk in the Kitchen*

Curiosity

Curiosity is a characteristic of all young creatures, but in none more developed than in the child. As Plutarch (46?–c. 120 A.D.) wrote long ago, "Children are much in love with riddles and such fooleries as are difficult and intricate; for whatever is curious and subtle doth attract and allure human nature as antecedently to all instruction agreeable and proper to it." Curiosity, an inquisitive insatiability, is the all-embracing trait of the child, for the child is interested in and curious about everything around him, and it is the trait that virtually leads to everything. There is no more permanent or certain characteristic of a vigorous mind than an unquenchable curiosity. Thomas Hobbes (1588–1679) put the case for curiosity admirably. In his book *Leviathan* (1651) he wrote, "The desire to know why, and how, curiosity, which is a lust of the mind, that by a perseverance of delight in the continued and indefatigable generation of knowledge, exceedeth the short vehemence of any carnal pleasure."

There are some who may not wish to go so far in celebration of curiosity, but fortunately we are not faced with a choice of alternatives, for both the short vehemence of carnal pleasures and the pleasures of the extended vehemence of curiosity both remain open to us.

Hobbes very rightly put the emphasis on the delight to which curiosity leads in the generation of knowledge. The satisfaction of curiosity is indeed among the greatest of pleasures. Curiosity is life, and without it life is impoverished and depleted. One must never, for whatever reason, turn one's back on life. If there ever was a neotenous trait more, almost, than any other, that must be kept alive and constantly exercised it is curiosity. New interests give one new life, infusions of vital spirits that keep one ever young, and a safeguard against boredom.

The Sense of Wonder

"The sense of wonder," writes Edith Cobb, "is spontaneous, a prerogative of childhood. When it is maintained as an attitude, or a point of view, in later life, wonder permits a response of the nervous system to the universe that incites the mind to organize novelty of pattern and form out of incoming information." Cobb goes on to point out that the ability of the adult to gaze upon the world with wonder is both a technique and a skill that are indispensable to the work of the poet, the artist, and the creative thinker. The sense of wonder is the beginning of all knowledge and of philosophy. It is a kind of exaltation of interest to which a certain excitement attaches, and which is accompanied by an expectation of "more to come," "more to do," the power of perceptual participation in the known and unknown.

It is this sense of wonder that leads the baby to discovery of his hands, nose, lips, genitals, fingers and toes, to the greater part of his body, and to that whole theater of perception that is the world he comes to know.

Wonder is associated with an elation that leads to that other trait that is so conspicuous a mark of the child, namely curiosity. The sense of wonder is a quality we never lose; what we do lose when that sense has been inadequately exercised is the extent of the landscape to wonder at, the ability to satisfy our wonder with the creative responses that would follow. It is difficult as an adult to make substantial advances in this quality, for it is a habit of mind that functions spontaneously and most easily when its cultivation has been early and prolonged.

Playfulness

Perhaps the best insight into the nature of play is that provided by Plato in *The Laws,* the book of his old age. The model of true playfulness Plato saw in the need of all young creatures to *leap*. And as Erik Erikson points out, "To truly leap you must learn to use the ground as a springboard, and how to land resiliently. It means to test the leeway allowed by given limits; to outdo yet not escape gravity." Hence, there is always a surprising element in play, transcending mere repetition or habituation, "and at its best suggesting some virgin chance conquered, some divine leeway shared." Erikson rightly notes that "what seems to become of play as we grow older depends very much on our changing conceptions of the relationship of childhood to adulthood and, of course, of play to work." Adults are inclined to judge play as neither serious nor useful, something unrelated to the center of human tasks and motives, and from which the adult, in fact, seeks "recreation." In a culture, however, such as that of the United States, in which adults have transformed play into an aggressive drive to win, in which on a frightening and festering scale sports have been degraded into big business, where even in our colleges and universities the coach is often the highest-paid member of the faculty, the authentic meaning and purpose of play has been confused and corrupted. Hence most of us come to have the most distorted view of play—*even* as recreation. Too many men take their recreation far too seriously, and instead of playing a game for the pleasure of it, play as if they were engaged in a deadly contest either with their "opponent" or with themselves, for at any cost they must win.

Man, especially in the "highly civilized" Western world, is the only creature who plays in this manner. All other creatures, including nonliterate peoples and most peoples of the non-Western world, such as the non-Westernized Chinese and Japanese, with few exceptions, play for fun, for the pleasure taken in the exhibition of skill and sportsmanship.

Animals when they play exult in the sheer pleasure of their romping and running, their mock chasing, waylaying, and biting each other. There appears to be little or no element of competition or hostility in their play—it seems sheer joy, and yet it is more than that. It is clearly a training and preparation for the challenges and realities of the adult world they will have to meet and to which they will have to make appropriate responses. The play of children is essentially of the same nature as that of young animals, but the child is capable of a far wider range of play activities than is any other creature, for the child's play is a *leap* of the imagination far beyond the capabilities of other creatures. It is this vaulting capacity of the imagination in play that is one of the most valuable traits of the human species. It is this sort of play of the imagination, the challenge to "take a giant leap," that has been responsible for much of the invention and discovery, the great ideas that have benefited humanity.

When we speak of "the poetic imagination," "the novelist's imagination," "the literary imagination," and the like, what we are really talking about (in addition to the hard work) is the frolicking, the leaping, the *play* of the imagination, of ideas and images of every kind. It is much the same kind as and in the direct line of descent of the play of the child. It was Nietzsche who said, "In the true man there is a child concealed—who wants to play."

We not infrequently hear someone who has completed what seems to us a preternaturally difficult task say that it was "child's play"—thus implicitly, if unconsciously, recognizing what had actually been involved in the accomplishment. The truth is that many people are engaged in activities that *are* "child's play" to them. From my own experience I would say that for most scientists their "work" has been but a continuation of their play as children. The play aspect of their work has been often acknowledged by scientists and other creative individuals.

The trick in life is to find something one enjoys doing and to make that one's way of earning a living. This can be greatly

facilitated by parents and teachers helping the young to cultivate their aptitudes and strengthen their weaknesses. But whatever occupation one is in, the element of play can always be
introduced to make a game of it—usually much to the improvement of the work and the pleasure one takes in it.

Genuine play is at its best when it is not restricted to the
attainment of a particular goal. In this kind of play one plays "for
the fun of it." And it is precisely such play that has led to the
enormous broadening of perceptual horizons, new discoveries,
further exploration, and mastery over the environment. Play has
probably been the most important factor in the evolution of social behavior among vertebrates, and as distinguished biologist
William H. Thorpe has remarked, probably also of the mental
and spiritual life of humankind.

Play is, of course, among the clearest of neotenous behavioral
traits. The ability to play is one of the principal criteria of mental
health.

Imagination

As a result of twenty years of research, including extensive
fieldwork, Edith Cobb concluded that a major clue to mental as
well as psychological and psychophysical health lies in the spontaneous and innately creative imagination of childhood. This she
saw both as a form of learning and as a function of the organizing
powers of the nervous system.

Childhood is the province of the imagination; yet in the waste-
land between imagination and reality only too often lie the un-
realized dreams of the child. Reality defeats most men, and only
a few dare challenge it with their imagination.

What is imagination? It is the power of forming mental images of what is not actually present, or the power of creating
mental images of what has never been experienced.

The imaginativeness of much of children's play, whether alone
or with others, whether of the "let's pretend" variety or some
other, is in the direct line of ascent to the scientist's "as if"
fiction, "let's pretend." The scientist says to himself, "Let me
treat this 'as if' it worked this way, and we'll see what happens."

He may do this entirely in his head or try it mathematically on paper or physically in the laboratory. What he is doing is using his imagination in much the same way the child does. The truth is that the highest praise one can bestow on a scientist is not to say of him that he is a fact-grubber but that he is a man of imagination.

And what is imagination really? It is play—playing with ideas. As the child replied when she was asked what she did when she made a drawing, "First I think, and then I draw a line round my think." A good deal of the time that is what we are doing as adults when we are imagining: "drawing lines round our thinks." Roger Fry, who asked the question of the little girl, believed that when left to themselves children never copy anything they see or draw from nature, but express with a delightful freedom and sincerity the mental images that make up their own imaginative lives. The imagination of the child creates its own reality, and that is, of course, what the creative artist does, whether he be poet, painter, sculptor, actor, dancer, musician, or novelist. It is also what the great scientist does, and it is to a considerable extent what each of us can do, for the faculty of imagination is never lost. All art speaks to us in the language of the imagination. It is not simply that the creative artist does what no one else has done before, but that he gives us, through the alembic of his imagination, a version of reality that would otherwise have been outside the range of our perception.

A certain painter, not without some reputation, early in this century defined "the art of painting" as "imitating solid objects upon a flat surface by means of pigments." He was quite serious. It is akin to Carlyle's description of the effects produced by a violinist as scraping upon the intestines of a cat with the hairs of a horse's tail. There are some people who go around the world and find it flat. Like our quoted painter, such people appear to be lacking in imagination, for it is what you bring to your experiences that infuses them with meaning—and that is what the great artist does in any medium.

It is the quality of the imagination that makes the difference between good and bad and indifferent art. Whether it be in painting, writing, music, or any other form of art, those who attempt to make the understanding do the work of the imagination are

unlikely to produce great art. It is the imagination that for the
most part gives us our originality. The repetitive clichéd existence of the unimaginative mind is a bore, and the conversation
of such persons, like their lives, is platitudinous, dull, dreary,
and disappointing, for the imagination is creative, and gives
color, freshness, and wit to our lives. There are those who can
turn a platitude into an epigram, and others who can turn an
epigram into a platitude. "Tell me, where is fancy bred?"

Take, for example, the way in which most people speak: They
speak in clichés, in stereotypes. It sounds like a dull routinized
series of chopped-up, all-too-familiar segments of sound, usually
pallidly inconsequential, wholly lacking in color, depth, originality, or wit—in short, noise. Noise is unwanted sound. Speaking is one of the most important things we do in our lives. Many
of us do not have enough imagination to realize that it is a great
art, which it is worth taking considerable pains with—not simply
because it is an art, but because it is a means of addressing the
humanity in us all, and art is the conquest of imagination over
time.

Children are especially good at original and imaginative use of
language. Some years ago the four-year-old grandson of a student of mine, having been given an explanation of what an anthropologist is and does in preparation for a visit by me, put to
me the following question in the course of that visit: "Why is
it," he asked, "that sometimes when I sit still for a long time my
leg begins sparkling?" Now that, I submit, is a much more accurate description in one word of what one's leg feels like than
saying it has "fallen asleep," and much more imaginative. He
had a second question for me: "Why is it when I am growing I
don't hear myself grow?" A splendid question, for if we were to
amplify what is going on during growth we would undoubtedly
be able to hear a great many sounds of different kinds. The point
is that this four-year-old thinker had used his imagination and
concluded there must be some noise during growth. What puz-
zled him was why he couldn't hear it. It is puzzles, questions
such as these that are the life-blood of science, philosophy, and
the active, imaginative mind in every area of life. The dimension
of the imagination is a highly enriching aspect of human existence, and an indispensable instrument in the interpretation of

reality. To dream, to fantasize is to have a vision that often exceeds the bare outlines of reality and creates a richer, more beautiful, more authentic reality than would otherwise be possible. Perhaps the best example of this is music; great architecture is another—as someone has said of King's College Chapel at Cambridge, it is music in stone. Imagination realizes what realism obscures or bungles. All great art, all great thought and deeds provide outstanding examples of the power of the imagination not only to transcend reality but to transform and create it anew. As Professor Jerome Singer put it in his study of the child's world of make-believe,

> What is perhaps most truly human about man, what is perhaps his greatest gift in the evolutionary scheme and indeed his greatest resource in his mastery of the environment and of himself, is his capacity to fantasize. To dream makes it possible to examine the alternatives that inhere [in] every moment as we organize our immediate experience. To be able to make-believe gives both the child and the adult a power over the environment and an opportunity to create one's own novelty and potential joy.

In the child's imagination lies the power to know and to create an environment, his own reality, and so it is with adults—those of us who continue to use our imaginations, for if you will keep your dreams, and dream new ones, you will never grow old.

Creativity

Childhood is the period of maximum creativity. During this period the child weaves his multiple experiences into a pattern that becomes himself. This self-creative process derives from the variety of experiences available to him in his encounter with and response to the environment, the wordless dialectic between himself and the world of his earliest days and years. In this encounter the child actively participates in the making of himself by creating mutual relations with the environment. This gives structure and function to the subsequent development of controlled perception and disciplined thought—"disciplined" in the sense that it becomes verifiable by the test of the environment or by the recollection of it. It is to soar with imagination into new realms of experience. From a very early period in his development the child ceases to be, if he ever was, a passive receiver of the messages transmitted to him from the environment, and becomes instead an enthralled creator, a molder and modeler of that environment, to the extent that he is permitted or assisted to do so by his socializers. A peculiar elation marks the child's response to the world, which is so new and exciting to him.

The child's need to live, to breathe, to be, to extend himself in time and space is stimulated by the challenges of virtually everything that impinges upon him. The world he constructs from virtually all that he absorbs and assimilates is constantly creative and renewing. Let no one ever think of the infant and child as passive recipients of the communications they receive, for they are anything but that. The creative capacity with which this marvelous creature is endowed is one of the many neotenous behavioral traits that have been overlooked as a constituent part of the endowment of every infant.

The qualities of creativity revealed in the studies of various investigators are virtually all present in the infant and child in, of course, a less sophisticated form. It will be useful to survey these briefly.

J. P. Guilford and his colleagues have recognized two different processes in thinking, namely the *convergent* and the *divergent*. In convergent thinking one comes up with an answer that is rather specifically implied by the nature of the information given, as, for example, two plus two equals four. In divergent thinking the individual generates a novel response or responses to the stimuli received. It has been found that convergent thinkers of both sexes, and all ages, tend to be conformists, and many more are found among those who enter the sciences than those who enter the arts; the latter tend on the whole to be divergent thinkers.

The qualities characterizing divergent thinking are also characteristic of creative types, and were largely derived from studies of adults and young people. Divergent thinking is also characteristic of infant and child, although, of course, in much less culturalized form. In the adult these processes are the trained development of the capacities of the child, and have become, therefore, abilities. Here are the subprocesses of divergent thinking:

Spontaneous flexibility, the ability to vary one's ideas over a wide range, even though it is not specifically called for, to produce a variety of possible answers to a problem rather than a restrictive one, or one limited to a single category.

Adaptive flexibility, the ability to vary one's ideas widely when the challenge of the situation requires it.

Redefinition, the ability to relinquish old ways of construing familiar objects in order to use them for a new purpose.

Originality, the ability to make unique or unusual responses.

Ideational fluidity, the ability to generate ideas quickly that will fulfill particular requirements.

Word fluency, the ability to generate words that fulfill particular structural requirements, such as providing as many words as possible that begin with a certain letter, or solving anagrams. The infant does this quite early with the babbling he develops, as well as with a whole range of meaningful sounds he attaches to feelings and objects.

Associational fluency, the ability quickly to generate words that meet particular requirements for meaning, such as providing a word that has about the same meaning as, for example, "good," or words meaning the opposite of "hard." Infants, in their own way, can probably approximate something like this, too.

There is, of course, a great deal more to say on the processes of creativity, but the criteria set out above should be sufficient for our purposes, which have a double aim: first, to underscore the fact that the essential processes of divergent thinking, of creativity, are already present in rudimentary form in the infant, and second, to make clear what the processes of creativity are, so that they may be more conscientiously encouraged, in the development of children, by adults who are not too far gone in their addiction to convergent thinking.

A multiplicity of different researchers have shown that achievers in later life have been strikingly of the divergent thinking type. Divergent thinking is a far better predictor of creativity than are IQ scores.

Make-believe and daydreaming are childhood traits that are of universal distribution, and there probably never has been an adult who has not indulged in this imaginative behavior—which is something more than imaginative, for it is very often creative (not that imagination isn't often also creative). One would be hard put to it to determine where, indeed, imagination ceases and creativity begins. The work of the imagination and creativity are not really separable activities, except insofar as creativity tends to be more structured and to lead more often to practicable results. Perhaps the most outstanding example of imaginative creativity, the product of daydreaming, is recounted by Friedrich August von Kekulé (1829–1896), German chemist. He achieved imaginative visualization of the structure of hydrocarbons during a reverie while seated atop a London bus; some years later, seated before a fire during a visit to the city of Ghent in Belgium, he fell into a doze, and the structure of the benzene ring came to him. Many creative spirits have testified to the importance of daydreaming and make-believe in their lives. As Charles Kettering (1876–1958), engineer, inventor, and President of General Motors Research Corporation, remarked, "Nothing ever built arose to touch the skies unless some man dreamed that it should, some man believed that it could, and some man willed that it must."

Studies on children who fantasize and daydream uniformly show that they rank much higher in creative storytelling and in the use of play equipment than those who do not. Interestingly, there are indications that the children with minimum daydream tendencies are likely to manifest signs of fixations or deprivation of such part-functions as orality (gratification from stimulation of the mouth area), diffuse aggression, or rejection. From other studies it has been found that creative young people, especially in artistic activities, have indulged in more imaginative play activities and daydreaming as children than have non-achievers.

Daydreaming and make-believe are often discouraged by parents in the mistaken belief that such activities represent mere idling and are in no conceivable way contributory to the welfare of the child. In this they are quite mistaken, unless, of course, these activities become an excessive substitute for the "real" world—and who is to say what may in any particular case be "excess"? The view that complete freedom or "permissiveness" affords the child the best opportunity for development is equally mistaken. Freedom is the most demanding of all responsibilities, and like every responsibility it is something that must be learned. Development is creative in the sense that it requires the work of the imagination and each of the faculties to give meaning and structure to its perceptions, and permits the child to move beyond the limited range of "real" experiences available to it.

Play, imagination, make-believe, daydreaming, reverie, and fantasy are fundamental neotenous traits that are precursors of creativity in young adult and later life. These represent the primary bases not only of creativity but also of the esthetic sense, as well as of creative scientific and artistic expression and appreciation. These precursors are the basic source of our delight in the adult make-believe of the theater, ballet, movies, games, art, poetry, style in every shape and form, the novel, short story, criticism, and every manner of esthetic experience. During such experiences we lose ourselves in the make-believe of the medium, becoming a part of it, and in this way the distractions of reality are for the time being dissolved. These are experiences we often recollect with pleasure in moments of tranquility. The yearning for such experiences is what makes art, science, philosophy, and the entertainment industry possible. But what in addition it makes possible is a fuller appreciation and enjoyment of life.

Hence, the implications of all this should be fully understood and recognized: the importance of the sociodramatic experiences in the life of the child continue into the life of the adult. This, in practical terms, mandates the encouragement of the sociodramatic activities in the very young child especially, and also in the classroom, in which the make-believe abilities of the child can be put to effective use, and classroom activities can be made through this means a great deal more appealing than they usually are. As Professor Jerome Singer has put it, "The use of less formal make-believe settings as part of the instructional procedure with children improvising skits about content material being studied in the classroom undoubtedly will enhance their interest and the positive affect associated with school, but also will help generate greater elaborative skills in communication as well." As Professor Singer observes, such activities have been found to be especially worthwhile for children from lower socioeconomic backgrounds, for whom the novelty and excitement of being a part of a dramatic production are morale building.

Putting oneself in the place of the other is a skill that plays a highly important role in successful social relations. Clearly this is an ability to which make-believe—for which "role-playing" is often another name—makes a very substantial contribution to social relations, and to what we call "thoughtfulness" and "sympathy." The creativity and make-believe behaviors in fashioning personal social skills can scarcely be overemphasized. Recognition of this fact has implications of the profoundest importance for child-rearing and education, and for the re-education of the adult. In the case of adults the adoption of the adult form of make-believe, the "as-if" principle—believing, in short, "as if" we were in fact what we ought to be and are now striving to be—can literally work miracles. By acting the role, for example, of a loving person, an unloving person can become a genuinely loving one—but only if, like the child, he believes in his make-belief. And every adult should, because such make-believe has the power to create him anew.

Each person by virtue of the fact that he is unique attempts a great deal of the time to renew himself by acts of personal creation, even while he is responding to the challenges of the environment in his customary, habitual manner—and I use both "customary" and "habitual" deliberately. I do this to underscore the fact that it is possible to break through the customary ways in which one has been conditioned and the habits one has formed, which have become second nature. The ability to modify, to change, to re-create oneself is the mark of the species to which we belong, and it is a mark of health. As René Dubos has said, "Health in the case of human beings means more than a state in which the organism has become physically suited to the surrounding physicochemical conditions through passive mechanisms; it demands that the personality be able to express itself creatively."

It should always be remembered that emotions are extraordinarily accurate sources of information, and that listening to them is often more revealing than the spoken word. Listening to emotions, our own and others', is a form of communication in which we resonate to the needs of others as well as to our own.

> . . . all that, lost beyond the reach of thought
> And human knowledge, to human eye
> Invisible, yet liveth to the heart.

The conclusion to which all the relevant research leads is that creativity is, if one must make a comparison, superior to mere intellectual activity, and, as Edith Cobb has said, we must learn to look at creativity from the viewpoint of value systems other than intellectual achievement.

As several investigators have agreed, the dimension of the unreal in human experience constitutes a critical feature of humankind's ultimate reality. We know that the unreal for innumerable human beings can be very much more real than the real; that the highly developed ability to fantasize is perhaps one of the criteria that differentiate humans from all other creatures, and is to be counted among the most valuable adaptive traits of our species. As Singer has pointed out, to dream makes it possible to examine the alternatives with which virtually every moment challenges us as we organize our immediate experience. "To be able to make-believe gives both the child and the adult a power over the environment and an opportunity to create one's own novelty and potential joy."

Finally, the world of make-believe leads to that creativity that comes from the striving to realize the possibilities of the dream.

Openmindedness

Among the most important of the child's traits is his openmindedness, his openness to every new stimulus that comes along. It is one of the loveliest things in the world to observe the freedom, the reciprocity, the willingness, without prejudice, with which the child receives and evaluates the world of excitements that impinge upon him. It is this freedom to accept every experience without prejudging it and to evaluate it for itself that is a heuristic neotenous behavioral trait, the potentialities of which are greater in humans than is even remotely approached by any other creature. The child's evolutionary striving is to connect every sensation with a meaning, and the culture into which he is born constitutes an adaptive zone of experience that serves to condition the meanings with which he endows such sensations as he is able to monitor. It is for this reason that to be born human is to be born in danger, for because of his openmindedness and lack of prejudice the child is always the victim of the prejudices of his socializers.

Openmindedness does not mean a mind so open that all critical judgment is suspended. But it does mean a mind that is open to all views and all experiences, a mind that is as free of prejudices as possible. And this is the kind of mind the child has and would continue to have and to develop were it not for the fact that in so many cases the environment into which he is born and "reared" is full of distorting socialization processes, which serve to close his mind and pervert his view of the world.

To the newness of the world the child brings an open mind; the adult, by contrast, only too often brings to the child's mind one that is closed, one that knows all the answers as well as *the* truth.

The neotenous sensibility of the child is directed toward growth in freedom, openness, and responsibility. And this, somehow, is perceived as a threat by most adults. Adults too often feel insecure unless they have fixed markers and artificial measures by which to categorize experience. The child, however, is naturally flexible because of his openmindedness and freedom from prejudgments. Jean Piaget, the eminent Swiss investigator of the growth and development of the child's mind, refers to *adaptation* as the most important principle in the development of mind. By adaptation Piaget means the continuous process of using the environment to learn, and learning to adjust to the environment. The process of adjustment consists of two complementary processes, *assimilation* and *accommodation*. Assimilation is the process of absorbing new information and fitting it into a preconceived notion about objects or the world. Accommodation means adjusting to new experiences or objects by revising the old plan to fit the new information. It is this dual process, assimilation-accommodation, that leads to adaptation, and enables the child to form new *schemata*—that is, mental images or patterns of action, a form of mental organization that enables the child to interpret the messages his senses deliver to him. And this is essentially the way in which the ability to think develops throughout life.

Adaptation seeks to establish a balance between the processes of assimilation and accommodation; this process Piaget calls *equilibration*. With the attainment of equilibration what stimulates the child to action are 1. the emotions that create the feelings that motivate learning; 2. differentiation of the nervous system, during which mental structures develop and the child becomes capable of greater understanding; 3. the exposure to a great variety of experiences through which the child can do his own learning and make his own discoveries; and 4. social transmission, or influential interactions with people, especially parents, teachers, and peers.

In the course of his development the child must sometimes unlearn various adaptations in order to make new ones, and this he begins to do at an early age. The progression from the thinking infant to the thinking adult is simply one of greater development of processes of thinking that are already at work in the infant. During this process of development many individuals are arrested at an infantile level, such as the *preoperational stage,* from two to seven years, in which the child perceives the world of people and things around him from only one point of view: his own. It is a phase of egocentricity in which the child perceives the world through mental images and symbols, which at this stage depend upon his own perceptions and his intuition. . . . And it is the age of curiosity, the never-ceasing questions, "Why, why, why?"—and the wonderings about adults, who quite clearly are not children, and who, it would sometimes seem from their behavior toward children, could never have been children themselves. The child's mind during this phase of his development has been beautifully sketched by Antoine de St. Exupéry in his classic book *The Little Prince*. The difference between the thought of the child and that of the adult is explained by the little Prince:

If I have told you these details about the steroid, and made a note of its number for you, it is on account of grown-ups and their ways. Grown-ups love figures. When you tell that you have made a new friend, they never ask you any questions about essential matters. They never say to you, "What does his voice sound like? What game does he love best? Does he collect butterflies?" Instead, they demand, "How old is he? How many brothers has he? How much does he weigh? How much money does his father make?" Only from these figures do they think they have learned anything about him.

Here the paedomorphic sensibility of the child is seen as early established. Interest in numbers comes with his growing ability to deal with concrete operations, from about ages seven to eleven. During this stage the child mainly deals with the present, the here and now. From ages eleven to sixteen the child thinks in formal operations, about the future, the abstract, and the hypothetical. During the adolescent period he thinks more flexibly, rationally, and systematically, and can look at a problem from different points of view. Openmindedness assumes a developed critical form, one that can operate on operations.

There is, of course, a great deal more to be said about the child's mental development, but here in this section we are concerned with his openmindedness, a subject that has received little if any attention from those interested in the development of children's behavior. Here we can do no more than emphasize the significance of openmindedness for the healthy development of every human being in every possible connection. The Greeks had a word for it, *eutrapelia*. It was the word Pericles used to describe the Athenians' lucidity of thought, clearness and propriety of language, freedom from prejudice and freedom from stiffness, their openness of mind, amiability of manners—all of which go along with a certain happy flexibility of nature.

It is toward the achievement of *"eutrapelia"* that all child-rearing practices and education should be directed, as well as all self-directed changes toward modification of the self.

Flexibility

Flexibility means to be pliable, malleable, supple, adaptable, and versatile, a trait or traits conspicuously characteristic of infant and child. It is a trait that is closely related to openmindedness, the need to learn, and to resilience, but is not quite the same. In the sense in which we generally observe the trait in children we may recognize one of its outstanding qualities in that polymorphous educability that enables the child to learn and acquire behaviors in response to any pattern of socialization to which he may be exposed. Behavioral flexibility is a species characteristic of humankind; no other creature remotely approximates that capacity for versatile response, for malleability. Flexibility is a quality of mind that is an invariable sign of mental health and humaneness. It is characterized by a willingness to listen to every cause and opinion, and to rethink one's basic beliefs in the light of new evidence, to exhibit an avidity for the growth and development of one's ideas and emotions, for the increase of our knowledge and the enlargement of our minds. It is to be alive and responsive to the new, and respectful of the old, to adjust and adapt to the challenge of new ideas, to guard against the development of prejudgments, to abhor all prejudices except those in support of truth, beauty, and goodness. To recognize the courage of their confusions in others, while not overlooking the possibility of them in ourselves, to be aware that the errors we are called upon to correct in others are exceeded only by those we are capable of committing ourselves, to grow and develop constantly in the qualities of our humanity; to share with Terence (*c*. 195–150 B.C.), the Roman playwright, the sentiment, "I am a man, nothing human is alien to me." It is the ability to identify oneself with others, to see and appreciate the differences, and to see the likeness in the differences; always remembering that differences are points of interest, that is never an argument against likenesses to point out the differences; that similarities are not as susceptible of definition as are differences.

It is not only flexibility in relation to others, important as that is, but also flexibility in relation to ourselves of which we must be constantly aware; to learn to combine tact and discretion with the courage of one's convictions, and never to trade with one's conscience, and always to make it a matter of conscience to be as well-informed as possible on those matters that call for one's attention; to know only one patriotism and one partisanship, namely to humanity.

Nor is it only to people that one's flexibility should be exhibited, but toward the whole world of nature, to inanimate nature as well as to all other living creatures. For all this children are abundantly prepared; they make little or no distinction between the animate and inanimate. Children are natural animists, they endow all things with living qualities, and set the example for adults.

Experimental-Mindedness

Young children are always experimenting. Adults are quite frequently unaware of the fact that children are born experimenters, and only too often attribute what should be quite clearly experimental behavior to something quite different. When, for example, a child pulls the wings off a fly it is often attributed to his innate naughtiness. When parents arrive home and find that Junior has taken the heirloom grandfather clock to pieces, it is ascribed to "the Old Nick in him." Such stereotyped reactions are unfortunate, wrong, and damaging. In pulling the wings off the fly or taking the clock apart the child is simply trying to discover how the creature works. How else can one do so? Poor Junior is entirely confused and dismayed to find that his perfectly natural impulse to discover how things are put together and how they work is rewarded with harsh and punishing behavior. It is very puzzling, very disheartening, and very unjust. But it is in the nature of Junior, of every child, to persist, and to try experiments that, if he is lucky, may not result in punishments. Such trials as he undergoes at the hands of his parents and/or socializers constitute, as it were, experiments in themselves, tests of adult toleration and even interest. And so, by trial and error, the child grows, in his ability to experiment, to test, in the art of checks and balances, costs and benefits. To play with toys and make them do one's bidding, to fantasize them into being what one wants them to be, and do what one wants them to; to float ships and send them off into some imagined seas opening on magic islands; to fly planes into space; to make toy boilers turn wheels and produce whistles; to experiment by dropping things into water, into holes; by walking in puddles with one's boots on; by knocking nails into pieces of wood; stuffing peas up one's nose, putting things in one's mouth to get the feel of them, lighting matches, and all the many other things of that kind that children do—all are experiments, and, of course, not all of them are to be encouraged! The consequences of stuffing peas up one's nose, playing with matches, and putting everything into one's mouth can be gently discouraged, if the child has not already sufficiently learned his lessons from the effects on himself of his experiments. When he is old enough to understand the risks and dangers they can be explained to him while his experimental interests are encouraged, for experimental thinking constitutes the best of all training in the ability to think soundly; that the child enjoys the opportunity to do so in interesting and practical ways is a boon that should be afforded him by all his socializers.

As a result of many investigations it has been established that from the earliest periods of childhood, culturally disadvantaged children show conspicuous developmental lag in such behaviors as transfer of objects from hand to hand, bimanual coordination, uncovering of hidden toys, and unwrapping of cubes. But even in culturally advantaged environments the value of encouraging the child's experimental-mindedness is often not understood. Bringing all his other capacities to bear on the world to which he must entrust himself—curiosity, imagination, openmindedness, creativity, playfulness, sense of humor, and creativity—the child arrives at his judgments in the best of all possible ways: by the experimental methods of verifiability and falsifiability, the very methods that are the basis of all science.

The standards that must be maintained in the development of scientific ideas necessitate the scrutiny and evaluation of assumptions; logic must be clear and faultless; facts must be verifiable; all the known facts must be accounted for; conclusions must follow from the evidence. All this, from the earliest ages, the child, in his own ways, is attempting to do, in his endeavor to make sense out of the world that is that larger womb into which he has been born.

The best thinking is almost always of an experimental nature—a setting up of hypotheses and a testing of them experimentally by their ability to withstand our best efforts at bringing them down. As I remarked earlier, good observation always contains an experimental element. Passive observation does not.

The good thinker is always experimental-minded, checking his observations as he makes them. As a consequence he always observes more and enjoys a fuller and wider range of experience than the non-experimental-minded individual.

The great innovators of the world, from prehistoric times to the present day, have all excelled in what they accomplished because they were the experimental-minded members of their society, who saw in their mind's eye new ways of doing things and new ways of solving old problems. Whether it was a new tool, a new habitation, or a new method of hunting, whether it was the development of language, social organization, art, music, counting, writing, reading, or any of the infinite number of innovations we have come to associate with civilization, it is the experimental mind we have to thank for these contributions.

Explorativeness

From the moment he is born—if he has not been drugged by poorly-informed obstetricians who have administered drugs to the mother during labor—the baby through all his senses immediately begins to explore the new world of experience before him. Through touch, vision, and hearing he embarks upon a voyage of exploration. Interestingly enough the word "explore" is derived from the Latin *explorare,* meaning "to search out," the word itself being derived from the affix *ex* meaning "out," and the word *plorare,* meaning "to cry out, to wail." This etymology suggests a profound understanding of the meaning of the newborn's first cry; in addition to being a bellows-like reflex action upon the inrush of air into the lungs, it may be perceived as a searching-out of the environment, essentially for the purpose of securing a response to his immediate need for a continuation of that comfort the baby so long enjoyed in the womb. Nothing is more calculated to elicit that comforting response from his mother than the baby's first cry. However that may be, the baby's almost immediate scanning of his mother's face, the exploration of every facet and expression of it, the investigation through touch of everything with which he comes into contact represent the forerunners of activities in which the child will engage as he grows older.

For the infant the world is a mystery, an unknown territory that must be explored and mapped. Mapping follows exploration, and by this means the child builds up the longitude and latitude and compass points of his relational world and gives it both pattern and form, by means of which he can negotiate his way through what gradually becomes for him a *terra cognita*.

The infant's discovery of his hands and arms, his fingers and toes, as he begins to sort them out from his angle of vision, to find that they belong to himself and can do his command, that fingers and toes can actually be a source of pleasure when sucked or nibbled on—all this conveys to him the unmistakable notion that exploration can in itself be a satisfying activity, one that can lead on to better and brighter things.

Scientific inquiry, research investigation, "finding out," and the like, all have their beginnings in the explorativeness of the child, a neotenous trait of supreme value, which is a never-failing mark of the active mind and the youthful spirit. Every original mind, in whatever field he or she works, is an explorer, and every active mind is engaged in some sort of explorative activity virtually every waking moment of the day. To be actively alive to the world in which we live means to be interested, involved, caring, and constantly alert and explorative. It matters not whether it be a novel, a biography, a painting, sculpture, poetry, or philosophy, or the solution of a problem, it is your active involvement in the process of exploration that will help to keep you growing young.

Resiliency

Resiliency is the ability to recover or bounce back from disturbing or distressing states induced by the external environment. The child possesses this ability to a quite astonishing degree. The younger he is the more resilient he appears to be. He can take all sorts of insults to his physical, physiological, and psychological well-being, as well as suffer massive deprivations of every sort, leading to very evident deficits and malformations, and rapidly recover from them in response to the restoration of healthy environmental conditions. There are innumerable instances of children of every age who, very near death from either disease, disorder, or lack of love, made spectacular recoveries in response to the appropriate measures. Others, almost as seriously affected, have come through as reasonably healthy persons in response to favorable changes in the environment. In a world in which a great deal of psychological anarchy has prevailed concerning the ability of the child to recover from damaging experiences, it is very necessary to emphasize this saving quality of resiliency, which constitutes one of the most valuable of the child's traits. Early deprivations are not irreversible, even though in many cases they may leave some evidence of their former presence.

Resiliency is characteristic of the fetus, and is a neotenous trait in infant and child, a trait that is conspicuously valuable in humans at all ages.

Like the good shock-absorbers on a car, which can take the bumps and roughness of the road, so, too, it is a great advantage to be able to take the stresses and strains in the course of daily life and bounce back as quickly as possible. As with all the other neotenous traits of the child, resiliency increases in strength and effectiveness with training—the training that the child's socializers should provide.

The Sense of Humor

As one who has been especially fond of babies from as early as he can remember, and who has been familiar with a large number of those delectable creatures, I have for many years been causing babies of six weeks of age or older to laugh till I have been forced to desist for fear of inducing an attack of hiccups. I induce the laughter or at the very least a smile by smiling broadly with lips that look like those of a clown, while simultaneously making gentle clucking sounds. This immediately attracts the attention of the baby, whose eyes soon light up. He either responds with a broad smile, and will continue to do so each time the clucking sound is repeated, or—more often than not—he breaks into unrestrained laughter. I mention this here because while I have done this with many infants, and rarely failed, I have never before published this observation. It is quite evident that babies as early as six weeks of age have a sense of humor, for they respond not merely to the sound and the face that goes with it but to the total configuration of both. They respond only to a face that is as smiling as it can be while engaged in inducing the response. Babies do not respond favorably to a frowning face. What is even more remarkable is that the same happy response can usually be induced in a baby who is crying. The smiling clucking seems to have a magical effect; a loudly crying baby on hearing it will suddenly stop crying, examine the sound-maker, and break into a smile. I imagine there may be other things capable of inducing the same response. Clearly, as the child grows the range of stimuli capable of making him smile or laugh enlarges. It is natural for children to laugh and to see the humor in all sorts of things, whether they be real, imagined, or of their own creation. They revel in the comic.

The development of that sense of humor is important, for without it life becomes a dreary business. It has been said that life for those who think is a comedy; for those who feel, a tragedy. To which it should be added that for those with a sense of humor it is a tragi-comedy. For it is the sense of humor that renders life a great deal more endurable than it would otherwise be, and much more amusing. Clearly humor is one of our greatest and earliest natural resources.

The sense of humor enlarges our perspective upon the world. And humor gives us an interior perspective upon ourselves. To be able to laugh at oneself is rather more valuable an accomplishment than the ability to laugh at others. It is the sense of humor about ourselves and about others that acts as a counter-balance to preserve our equilibrium, and that often has the power to assist others in preserving theirs. The ability to perceive what is funny, amusing, or ludicrous, in the somber and the serious as well as in the comic, adds greatly to the flavor of living, and constitutes a sovereign defense against the bores and the boring, the sedate and the solemn, the dreary and the dull.

One need not count that day lost during which one has not laughed, but that day is truly lost in which the play of one's sense of humor has not been given its appropriate exercise. Every day provides abundant opportunities to see and to respond to what we may alone perceive as funny, either about ourselves, things, or other people.

Playfulness and the sense of humor are, of course, very closely allied, as are laughter, wit, imagination, and creativity. It is in the play of ideas and the unexpected, the incongruous and yet strangely congruous, that humor is generated.

Joyfulness

One of the most neglected of all the traits of the child is his joyfulness. This is, of course, connected with his sense of humor, though the traits are quite distinct from each other. One can see the joy in the face and eyes of a small baby who has been loved and caressed into that security and trust he reflects, trailing clouds of glory, as Wordsworth put it:

> Blest the Babe,
> Nurs'd in his Mother's arms, the Babe who sleeps
> Upon his Mother's breast, who, when his soul
> Doth gather passion from his Mother's eye!
> Such feelings pass into his torpid life
> Like an awakening breeze, and hence his mind
> Even (in the first trial of its powers)
> Is prompt and watchful, eager to combine
> In one appearance, all the elements
> And parts of the same object, else detach'd
> And loth to coalesce.
>
> And, then, when he grew older,
>   in all things now
> I saw one life, and felt that it was joy.

And in joy the human is designed to grow and develop. The sorrows and setbacks that are incident to the human condition, the disappointments and bereavements one will inevitably suffer, must be accepted as well as we are able, while the "never-failing principle of joy" remains—that is, *should* remain. Unfortunately, joyfulness is not generally cultivated in children, and is a rather hollow prescription for those many children whose saddening and joyless daily lives seem to be beyond the reach even of consolation. Yet cheerfulness will keep creeping in.

One has only to observe the romping and sheer delight when children are playing together to know that joy, fun, is as strong a biological drive as any other. The child is naturally to joy inclined, and every normal child is born with the capacity for it, even with the capacity to generate it for himself. Still joy, like smiling and laughter, is essentially a shared experience, and is at its best when it is so. All joy is young, and age sets no boundaries to it. Yet in a great part of the Western world there has been a massive failure to recognize the importance of joy as a developmental need and a vital necessity. The very idea of "fun" has been corrupted and deformed, especially in the New World, in which the infection has assumed epidemic proportions. In America, as we know, children are taught to play games not for the joy of it but in order to win. Parents, teachers, coaches, and spectators all seem to be engaged in a conspiracy to take the joy out of games. The thing, on the contrary, is to be deadly serious, and never to give your opponent an even break, but to take advantage of every one of his weaknesses. The main thing is winning: "the name of the game," as the saying so aptly puts it. Outmoded, effete notions of sportsmanship are strictly for the birds. "First is first, and second is nowhere." Indeed, "games" and "sports" have become the highly remunerative grand highways to success and public adulation. "Sports" are now transmogrified into big business, parents training their children at very early ages to play tennis or baseball or whatever, in the hope that they may one day become champions and compete in domestic and international matches, which will enable them to win enormous cash prizes; they then will become multimillionaires before they reach their middle twenties.

The emphasis is on winning, not on doing your best and rejoicing in whoever may win, playing for fun and for the pleasure of meeting the challenges of the other so that the best is brought out in each. It is in such a manner both grow, and grow together rather than apart. A game becomes a *cooperatively* competitive *sport,* rather than a *competitively* competitive *conflict* in which the sole purpose is to win in order to reap the rewards of both acclaim and cash, and in which the loser slinks sullenly away, not infrequently hurling a few obscenities at referee, photographers, and spectators. The unsportsmanlike spectacles highly paid professional players have made of themselves in virtually all sports have set the most abject examples, especially for children. Were sports really understood for what they should be—training grounds for the development of character, the "good sport"— the professional yahoos who frequently disgrace themselves, especially on the tennis courts, would become a thing of the past. Playing a game comprises not alone the ability to play skillfully, but also the ability to enjoy it, to have fun, to do one's best, and to preserve and emulate those graces that are the mark of the civilized, the civil, mind; to extend to one's opposite number those civilities, that courtly behavior that should constitute the unwritten law of every game. For though it has been said often enough before, what really matters is not whether you win or lose, but how you play the game.

I deliberately speak of games in a section of "Joyfulness" rather than "Playfulness" because I think it important to draw the attention of the reader to an aspect of games and sports that is virtually threatened with extinction. I do not wish here to belabor the point, but I do desire to emphasize the importance of doing what needs to be done to bring up children to play games cooperatively, to encourage amateurism in sports, and to accomplish the complete discontinuance of professional sports of every kind. Where business enters into games they cease to be games, and suffer that corruption and degradation which is inevitably associated with their exploitation for money.

Laughter and Tears

The infant begins to smile and to laugh quite early in life. He is capable of smiling from the first day of birth; this is thought to be purely physiological or reflexive. Nonselective social smiling in response to a mobile human face develops around the eighth week. By nonselective one means that the infant will smile at a face with which it is not familiar as readily as it will with one that it is. At about the fifth or sixth month, selective social smiling develops. The infant now reserves his smiling for familiar individuals: parents, siblings, relatives, and primary caretakers. It has been established that the infant's readiness to smile will be increased by a socially responsive environment and decreased by a socially unresponsive one. All investigators agree that the infant's readiness to smile is produced by socially encouraging—that is to say, socially reinforcing—conditions.

Laughter, which generally emerges at about twelve weeks but in many cases earlier, also develops in relation to social situations. By the age of two years children tend to laugh most in response to motions made by themselves, and next in order at socially unacceptable situations. By three years of age the latter leads the former, and laughter occurs in response to grimaces and word play. Thereafter laughter is evoked by a multiplicity of stimuli.

Children of high intelligence generally laugh more than children of average or somewhat above average intelligence, as "measured" by IQ tests. It is, however, generally agreed that factors in the child's social and emotional history are likely to have a more important bearing upon his disposition to laugh than the factor of intelligence alone.

The joyful, ringing laughter of children is one of the pleasantest sounds to rejoice the human ear. At any age it is one of the most agreeable traits in any person. What Dante saw in Paradise was equal ecstasy, one universal smile of all things.

So children should be encouraged in that "sudden glory" that is laughter, for laughter is not only a social solvent, the smile a token of relatedness, but both are socially binding accomplishments that contribute to biological and social health, of both the individual and the group. That is why, at all ages, we so much value those who make us laugh, and are more ready to respond in a friendly manner to those who approach us with a smile.

> A friend approached me today,
> I had never met him before.
> We shared a lifetime of smiles.
> I never needed to ask what for.
> ANONYMOUS

Clearly the smile and the laugh are of great adaptive value, for they biologically facilitate the social interaction between persons.

Among some nonliterate peoples what we perceive as aggressive behavior in a child is generally met not with a reprimand or counteraggression, but with laughter and fun. We have already seen in a previous chapter how among the Fore of New Guinea, for example, what we view as aggressive behavior in a small child they perceive as a form of exploratory physical play. Aggressive behavior by a young child is typically received with amusement and affection. The toddler is never chastened or reproached, but engaged in diversionary activities, each occasion being made one for fun and laughter. The result is that the Fore have grown into quite remarkably healthily unaggressive persons. But, alas, civilization seems to have caught up with the Fore; now, having become coffee growers and traders, the Fore are no longer laughing as much as they once did, and competition and aggression are replacing the old ways. Thus do we bring the benefits of civilization to the "primitive" peoples of the world.

Human laughter is a defining trait of our species, just as weeping is, for humans are the only creatures who have the neurophysiological mechanisms for either, not to mention, as the cynic might remark, more cause to both laugh and weep than any other creature.

The age at which human infants begin to cry with tears varies considerably. Some infants are able to shed tears at or shortly after birth, others fail to do so until they are eight weeks old. The average age at which tears begin to accompany emotional weeping is between five and six weeks. The peak of the ability to weep is reached in infancy and childhood, between six and nine years, and gradually tapers off in adulthood. The late development of weeping in the human infant suggests that it is a trait that developed some time after assumption of human status and its accompanying prolonged period of dependency.

Optimism

Children are natural optimists, for the future appears to them to be suffused with promises that will surely be fulfilled with growth. That is why children are so impatient to grow up. And in the best of all possible worlds those promises *would* be fulfilled.

Children can only look forward to a future of grown-upedness, which appears to them so much more rewarding than being a growing child. It seems so interminably long before one will achieve grown-upedness. Most children carry with them the feeling that whatever the state of things "now," they can only improve with time. The child lives in a world of rising expectations, and because he does so he puts the self-fulfilling prophecy— when permitted—to constant good use. When he is optimistic about the outcome of anything he is likely to do the necessary to make it come true. Hence optimism serves a very real biological and social function: It enables the individual to realize himself as a person and at the same time to grow in socially useful skills, which are ultimately of benefit to the group. It is not simply somatic anticipations and neural expectancies in which infancy and childhood are enmeshed, but its functional capacities, both physical and behavioral, which the child looks to have satisfied. Under the circumstances the only possible tenable position for him to maintain is one of optimism that the promised rewards will be forthcoming. We are born optimistic, "trailing clouds of glory do we come," for no one strives more or is better prepared to live than the newborn. The happy child is the born optimist, and is clearly designed to employ his optimism as the magic vehicle that leads to fulfillment. Lionel Tiger, in his book entitled *Optimism,* has argued that optimism is not an optional trait but as natural to humans as eyes that see and as irreplaceable as air. I think he is right, that optimism is a neotenous trait that serves both biological and social functions of great value and importance. Tiger suggests that there is a neurophysiology for a sense of benignity of the future. Here, too, I believe the evidence does suggest that optimism exists because it is of great adaptive value, and that its physiological substrate is represented by internal secretions that affect the brain "in an optimistic manner."

Assuming a biological base, anything that militates against optimism is by definition maladaptive. Optimism contributes to mental, physical, and social health, and moreover puts one in a frame of mind for the achievement of ends that the pessimist regards as impossible. The optimist won't easily give up. The Wright brothers were told by the world's leading authorities that a heavier-than-air flying machine was both a mathematical and a physical impossibility. But they, who were only a couple of small-town bicycle mechanics, knew better. Their optimism was based on experimental results, which told them that with the solution of certain problems, especially in the design of wings, they might get such a machine into the air. It was their optimism, when no one else could see any sensible reason for it, that carried them to success. In spite of the fact that they had repeatedly flown their machine over a field outside Dayton, the Wrights were unable to interest newspaper reporters to come and see the miracle for themselves. The newspapermen later said they simply didn't believe that such a flying machine was possible.

The optimistic frame of mind is one that reinforces itself, for the optimist is constantly being reminded of the value of that trait by the frequency of his success. He develops confidence, confirming him in the belief that whatever he undertakes will prove successful, and although that does not always turn out to be the case, his confidence carries him through most of the time to successes that might not otherwise have been possible. Even in a time of doubt and crisis the optimist knows that the only philosophically tenable position even for a pessimist is optimism. Optimism is creative in the sense that it often leads to solutions of difficult problems and discoveries that could not have been made without it.

It is obvious that optimism and perseverance are closely allied, and that the first precedes the second, for without optimism as to the outcome there would be very few perseverers. Without such optimism Paul Ehrlich (1854–1915), the German biochemist, would never have discovered, after more than 600 trials, the effectiveness of salvarsan (and neosalvarsan after 914 experiments) in the treatment of syphilis; nor would Thomas Edison have discovered the successful material to serve as the filament for the electric bulb had he not had the patience to persist after innumerable unsuccessful trials with various will-o'-the-wisps. Many similar stories could be told; the reader is doubtless familiar with several. "It's dogged as does it" was Darwin's motto. A great part of the world of discovery and invention is due to the perseverance and optimism of the benefactors of humanity.

Another trait associated with the optimistic personality is enterprise. Not all enterprise succeeds, but this much is certain: Very few enterprises entered upon by a pessimist ever succeeded. The pessimist simply doesn't have the right approach.

These three traits—optimism, perseverance, and enterprise— are what make the world go round, contributing at every level of civilization to the greater comfort and happiness of humankind. They are traits that should be nurtured in every human being from infancy throughout life.

Honesty and Trust

My dictionary says of honesty that it is the state or quality of being honest, and it defines honesty as

> 1. orig., *a* held in respect, honorable, *b* respectable, creditable, commendable, seemly, etc.: an epithet or commendation 2. that will not lie, cheat, or steal; truthful; trustworthy 3. *a* showing fairness and sincerity; straightforward; free from deceit [an *honest* effort] *b* gained or earned by fair methods, not by cheating, lying, or stealing [an *honest* living] 4. being what it seems; genuine; pure [to give *honest* measure] 5. frank and open [an *honest* face] 6. [Archaic] virtuous; chaste.

The child is naturally all these things. The sincerity, straight-forwardness, trustfulness, and fairness of children, when they have not been deformed by a destructive "upbringing," are among their most striking traits. They, of course, require guidance in learning such things as that it is not always either necessary or desirable to tell people the truth about themselves, even when they want to know it; that frankness can often be in bad taste and damaging, and so on. We need to understand that when children lie, cheat, or steal, it suggests that the conditions that produced such behavior require looking into. The child has to learn to distinguish between the real and the unreal, that his world of make-believe, which seems to merge into reality, requires some differentiation. A great part of the make-believe world is often a wish-fulfillment and also at once a means of eliciting sympathy, as when a child announces to his friends that his cat or dog or sibling or parent has died. This is seen by adults as a lie, and from their point of view it may be, but it needn't be so to the child. Romancing, tale-telling, and deliberate distortions of the truth are part of the normal development of the child, and should be recognized for what they are: the novelistic capacities of the child, forerunners of the more developed abilities of an adult able to enchant the world with his story-telling. We see this novelistic element not only in the literatures of the world, written and unwritten, but also in works of art of every kind, which is a prime reason why the romancing, tale-telling, and make-believe of every sort should be treated with understanding, sympathy, and the helpfulness that enables the child to understand the difference between reality and unreality, between truth and untruth, as well as such moral issues as are within his comprehension.

It is because adults are so much exercised over what they take to be the ''naughty'' or ''bad'' behavior of children that they fail to perceive the essential honesty of the child. It is a revealing fact that one may look in book after book on child growth and development and not find a word relating to this conspicuous trait, the honesty of the child, not to mention many of the other characteristics of the child discussed in this book. I cannot think that the writers of such works have taken the child's basic honesty for granted. I rather think that in the attempt to gain experimental control and scientific rigor, laboratory studies tend to produce a narrow view of the child's behavior. Whatever the reason, honesty has been wholly overlooked. I suspect that this is also in part due to the fact that we all begin with preconceptions concerning the nature of the child and allow these to prejudice our view of it. Those who believe in the doctrine of original sin in any of its versions, religious or secular, will begin with the assumption that the child is innately depraved, and will act toward him accordingly, in this way vicariously realizing the self-fulfilling prophecy in the child. Subscription to the view that the child is ''sinful in the flesh'' has resulted in a focus and search for evidences of sin in the child; and what from such an angle of vision one is looking for, one is bound to find. Such a viewpoint has greatly prejudiced and influenced our conception of the parental role as the policeman whose function it is to punish and repress "bad" behavior, enforce the law, and teach the rules of "good" behavior.

Talk with teachers about the honesty of young children and I venture to say you will hear some surprising things. As one of them, my neighbor Julia Gordon, author of *My Country School Diary,* responded from her many years of experience with children in the classroom, "Of course they're honest," she said. "They see things as they are, and 'tell it like it is,' sometimes to the point of hurting, until they learn not to. When they 'make believe,' 'pretend,' they know very well what they are doing." Their honesty is not an acquired quality—that is the way they are.

The absolute honesty of the child is reflected in the behavior of the children of most nonliterate people. Many an anthropologist and traveler has had occasion to comment on this. As Francis Hutcheson remarked long ago in his *System of Moral Philosophy* (1755), "Truth is the natural capacity of the mind when it gets the capacity of communicating it, dissimulation and disguise are plainly artificial effects of design and reflection." As I have already observed, and as G. Stanley Hall, the great child psychologist, pointed out, children frequently regard every deviation from the most literal truth as heinous. In many children this fear of telling an untruth becomes an occasion for adding even to a simple "yes" or "no," either mentally, whispered, or aloud, "I think" or "perhaps." Those words were written in 1890, but they hold largely true for small children today.

Because loved and unfrustrated children seem to me to be naturally honest, I regard honesty as a neotenous behavior trait; as such the cultivation of the child's honesty constitutes a reinforcement of his mental health, as well as that of the health of his community.

Compassionate Intelligence

The perfectly natural compassion and intelligence of the child is seen in its solicitude and love for younger children and especially for small animals, as well as its solicitude for suffering of any kind. Compassionate intelligence has its origins in the maternal-infant relationship, a biological reciprocity, a cooperativeness, out of which all social relations grow. Compassionate intelligence is closely related to love, but is not quite the same thing. Compassion refers to deep sympathy and desire to help the sufferer, and if hard pressed, I would suppose it difficult in many instances to distinguish it from love; still, compassionate intelligence also implies something of pity, which is never present in love, and in addition to compassion there is the element of intelligence, the ability to make the most appropriately successful response to the particular challenge of the situation. In brief, then, compassionate intelligence is involvement in the other's plight combined with the desire to help in some practical way. Children exhibit this gift quite early, and should, of course, receive every encouragement to exercise it.

In the societies of the Western world compassionate intelligence is encouraged in girls—in boys it is tabu. The tabu on tenderness in which boys are conditioned, the emphasis on "manliness," "machismo," plays havoc with the male's capacity for compassionate intelligence. Tenderness is considered to be feminine, and that is sufficient to remove it from the repertoire of masculine behavior. Indeed, things have reached such a pass in the Western world that many men seem to have lost all understanding of its meaning. The masculine world would substitute for it the idea of "justice." The difficulty with that is that there is not much compassion in their justice, and justice without compassion is not justice at all. As Sir Thomas Noon Talfourd (1795–1854), the English jurist and dramatic poet, remarked, "Let us have just men on our benches, but not so just that they forget human frailty."

The world stands greatly in need of men and women who are both compassionate and intelligent. As Edith Cobb has written,

> If cultural attitudes could be shifted toward a recognition of human desire to exercise a compassionate intelligence, not only as tool and method but also as the chief human survival function, we would, I believe, find ourselves capitalizing on the human impulse to nurture, cultivate, and extend this vast potential. It is even conceivable that the economic motive, which at present dominates social structure, and stifles other styles of motivation, could be enlisted if all humanity's health and welfare were seen to be at stake.

Indeed, the knowledge is available, and techniques are known, by which this imprisoned splendor, this creative drive, could be released.

> Truth is within ourselves; it takes no rise
> From outward things, whate'er you may believe:
> There is an inmost centre in us all,
> Where truth abides in fulness; and around,
> Wall within wall, the gross flesh hems it in,
> Perfect and true perception—which is truth;
> A baffling and perverting carnal mesh
> Which blinds it, and makes error: and, *"to know"*
> Rather consists in opening out a way
> Whence the imprison'd splendour may dart forth,
> Than in effecting entry for the light
> Supposed to be without.
>
> ROBERT BROWNING
> *Paracelsus*

My reading of the evidence tells me that the directiveness, the striving, of the child is toward goodness, a longing that every human being at some time in his life experiences, and that in the truly healthy human constitutes the landscape, the background of his life. What the newborn commences with by way of human nature is good. It is not neutral, or indifferent, but good, good in the sense that the child is designed to grow in the ability to love. It is human nurture that distorts and confuses. The theories of Konrad Lorenz, Robert Ardrey, and others to the effect that humans are innately aggressive, are, in the light of scientific evidence, quite untenable. It is easy to attribute the evil behavior of some humans to "original sin," or, as our Victorian forebears so engagingly called it, "innate depravity." It is even easier to saddle "wild animals" with the evil conduct of which humans alone are capable, and then to "trace" our allegedly evil propensities back to our animal ancestry. It all seems to make sense, for how is the unsophisticated reader to perceive the circularity in the reasoning, especially when scientists who appear to be authorities set the "facts" before him? The answer to that question is, of course, that it isn't easy, especially when facts are wrenched out of context and are not what they seem to be. We in the Western world are part of a long tradition that has found the doctrine of original sin a congenial explanation for the horrors that have disfigured man's history. How else can one account for this bloody history, for the holocaust, for the crime, murder, sadism, and brutality of so many allegedly civilized people?

The answer is that in societies of the Western world we have deprived innumerable children of their birthright, the need for love, and subjected them to all sorts of deforming pressures. In the lands most guilty of these offenses against children the crime rates of every kind are the highest. Deprived children who have never learned how to relate to others grow up seeking to survive without involvement in the welfare of others, without thought or feeling for others, but with a deep craving for the love that has been denied them, and which they generally identify with power, respect, and success. They are the victims of a world they never made, of which tragically enough they become the chief proponents and the most powerful perpetuators. In their extreme forms they become criminals. When at last our so-called "civilized" societies come to understand these simple truths, we may look forward to a very different world, not one of perpetual conflict, brutality, alienation, and misunderstanding, but one of compassionate intelligence and peace . . . "and a little child shall lead them" (Isaiah, 11:6).

Dance

We have already referred to the evidence that children are born with a natural sense of rhythm. It is a sense that, there is some reason to believe, is developed in the womb, possibly in part as a consequence of the cradling and rocking of the fetus in co-oscillation with the mother's movements, and the syncopated response to the mother's heartbeat. The baby is already in tune with the deepest rhythms of existence. The dance of life has begun.

We have also discussed the recent research indicating that the newborn dances—that is, rhythmically responds—to speech by synchronizing his pattern of movement with speech. Drs. William S. Condon and Louis W. Sander of Boston University have described this rhythmic interaction between baby and mother as a subtle ballet. Such silent duets of body-language can only be picked up in careful analysis of film showing the interacting couple projected in slow motion. Similar balletic movements usually become apparent in scenes between children, and also in social settings among adults.

It is fascinating to watch children of two or three years, either spontaneously or in a social situation where others are dancing, break out into a dance in perfect rhythm to whatever kind of music may be playing. I have seen a three-year-old American white girl dance to a record that yielded the dance music of some ten different cultures, from African and American Indian to Zulu. The astonishing thing about her performance was that although she was not observed to have danced before this occasion, she spontaneously changed dance styles in complete harmony with each change of ethnic music. I have heard of similar performances, but this one I witnessed myself.

It was astonishing, because the child had not previously heard such music, and so far as I know had never seen anyone dance in any style whatever. Yet she responded with perfect dance movements to the music she heard. When, for example, a Hopi Kachina dance was played, she did a perfect Kachina dance, with arm, leg, and body movements that would have delighted and met with the approval of any Hopi. Yet in later life she never danced.

The relationship between music and dancing is profound, for it is the music that determines the purposeful intentionally rhythmical and culturally patterned sequences of nonverbal body movements. Many folk songs are conceived as inseparable from dancing. Musical form, as for example the rondo (round dance), has often been shaped by dance form. It is possible to dance without music, but that is usually to a cadence created by the dancer to his own beat.

Dancing is clearly a behavioral trait that children delight in. Indeed, in some cultures it is the dancing of children that sets the pattern for the dances of the adults. Among the Dagomba of Northern Ghana, for instance, children learn social habits and personal discipline through music and the dance. There it is the children who plan the music, songs, and dances. Through these means the young people are often able to express their ambivalence about the world in which they are growing up, and through their provocative, humorous songs and dances to say much that could not be otherwise expressed. In this way, as the elders acknowledged, children give meaning to tradition. As one Dagomba said,

> If you want to see our way of life, you will see it from the children. Even when we watch them play, and we watch how often they are with each other, we know how they will end up. So it is the children who make our culture, because the children can do something and it will come to stand as something for the old people. All our old dances, the children didn't start them, but when children play, they dance them. And the new dances we have not seen before, it is the children who started them, and when these children grow up, these dances will become an old thing to them. And so, for our way of life, it all starts from the children.

What a contrast to the Western world's way of slighting the contributions children are capable of making! At one time singing and dancing were encouraged in our schools. The encouragement is no longer as enthusiastic as it once was.

Early in this century the great American educator G. Stanley Hall deplored the decline of dancing as part of the educational experience in the schools. He urged that it was imperatively needed to give poise to the spirit, schooling to the emotions, strength to the will, and to harmonize the feelings and the intellect with the body that supports them. Plato, in the final work of his old age, the *Laws,* declared that a good education consists in knowing how to sing and dance well. "Of dancing," Plato wrote,

> there is one branch in which the style of the Muse is imitated, preserving both freedom and nobility, and another which aims at physical soundness, agility and beauty by securing for the various parts and members of the body the proper degree of flexibility and extension and bestowing also the rhythmical motion which belongs to each, and which accompanies the whole of dancing and is diffused throughout it completely.

It is most desirable that dancing be restored to its proper place in the school curriculum. Its abandonment in many schools at a time when the enthusiasm of the young for every form of dance has reached an all-time high, in the period, that is, from the Jazz Age in the twenties to the Disco of the seventies and eighties, is surprising. Things have so far advanced that in the eighties there are entrepreneurs still in high school who have opened and successfully run discotheques for teenagers.

It is not only children and teenagers who love to dance; so do adults. However, many adults seldom or never dance. It is not encouraged in Western societies, except on special occasions. Indeed, dancing by the old is strongly discouraged by the young. Young people have an extraordinary dislike for seeing anyone over forty on the dance floor. They seem to feel that dancing in older people is unbecoming, that it is "out of place," the proper place, presumably, being somewhere out of sight. Adults in their forties are barely tolerated, but certainly dancing adults beyond fifty are regarded with distaste as having committed something resembling a breach of good manners.

With the greater understanding of the young for older people such attitudes will become truly anachronistic. Meanwhile, whatever age one may be, one should dance, and dance frequently, for there are few activities so wholly and deeply gratifying. A partner, though desirable, isn't always necessary; dancing by oneself doesn't mean that one is really dancing alone. One should remember that much of ballet dancing is solo, and so may be any other form of dancing.

Dancing can be viewed as a graceful cadence of the body through movement in harmony with the music. Dance, indeed, is the language of movement. The great joy of dancing derives from the elegance and improvisation with which one moves virtually every movable part of one's body. By improvisation I mean the individual inventiveness one brings to the dance, however formally structured it may be. One must allow the music to enter one's bones, to respond to it with all the faculties it calls for, for it is an art of many sensory dimensions. As Havelock Ellis wrote in his delightful book *The Dance of Life* (1923), "Dancing is the loftiest, the most moving, the most beautiful of the arts, because it is no mere translation or abstraction from life; it is life itself."

It is, indeed, the very rhythm of life. Can anything be more exhilarating than a beautiful ballet? I had the good fortune to see the original Diaghilev ballets in London during the early twenties. I have been nourished by that experience all the days of my life—the genius of the dancers, the marvelously original décor, such sets as only a Picasso could dream up, the music of Stravinsky, of Tchaikovsky, the color, the lighting, the production, the incredible opulence of it all combining to create so beautiful an enrichment of life. Diaghilev, *"ce prodigeux animateur"* who made it all possible, was fiercely unwilling to settle for anything less than the best and pluperfect, down to the last detail.

The experience of dancing constitutes something more than a body in motion. There is a release and a replenishment of psychic energy that leaves one with an oceanic feeling of freedom from which all constraint has fallen away, in which the free play of the emotions in disciplined response to the music has its way. One is infused with a lyrical joy. Little wonder that such feelings have been perceived as reminiscent of the nurturance and protection of the prenatal and infancy stages. However that may be, and whether one dances by oneself or with others, it is the positive reinforcements that one receives from this poetry of motion, this feeling of being in tune with the universe, that is so uplifting and constructively beneficial. It would be difficult to think of any activity of greater therapeutic value.

In addition, dancing is one of the best forms of exercise for both the body and the soul. Interestingly enough, it appears to have been esteemed from the earliest times. Dancing, as Plato said, concerns the body, and music aims at goodness of soul.

Song

Who any longer sings? Not so long ago almost everyone did. Before the advent of television—that is, before we became a watching society and learned to sequester ourselves from each other in the same room—the family would gather round the piano, sheet music was inexpensively available, and the whole family sang. No longer. Today, singing is for professionals, with the young as their principal supporters, for it is to them that the lyrics and the music are specifically addressed. The lyrics express their feelings, their longings, and their dissatisfaction with the way things are. However well some of these modern troubadours may express their feelings, the young, like their elders, would be better served were they to learn to sing for themselves, and if they felt like it create their own lyrics, just as so many other peoples do.

And, of course, everyone should be taught to play a musical instrument. Many schools do provide such teaching, and some of our greatest musicians have first learned to play their instruments at school. It is not, however, the production of great musicians that our schools should aim to achieve, but rather a basic ingredient of every liberal education, namely a competence in the art and practice of music. Music is the universal language of humanity, and utters the things that cannot be spoken. To be able to make music, whether by voice or instrument or both, is the most gratifying and solacing of experiences.

> Music, the greatest good that mortals know,
> And all of heaven we have below.
>> JOSEPH ADDISON
>> *Song for St. Cecilia's Day*

When one is becalmed music has the power to give wind to our sails, and

> Where griping griefs the heart would wound
> And doleful dumps the mind oppress,
> There music with her silver sound
> With speed is wont to send redress.
>> RICHARD EDWARDES
>> *A Song to the Lute*

Children are natural singers, hummers, and dancers. Let us encourage them in these arts, and let us continue to sing, dance, and be merry, as long as we are able.

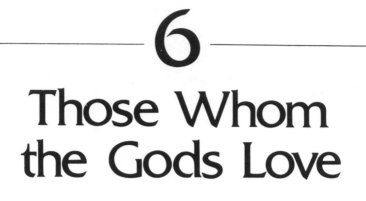

Those Whom
the Gods Love

Grow young along with me!
The best is yet to be,
The last of life, for which
    the first was made.
                    —AMENDED AFTER ROBERT BROWNING
                    Rabbi Ben Ezra

It was Oscar Wilde, that splendid philosopher, who, improving
upon Menander, observed that those whom the gods love grow
young. It is quite true. Wilde perfectly understood that the gods
love those who grow young because they have taken the trouble
to be so. The youth of the chronologically young is a gift; growing young into what others call "old age" is an achievement, a
work of art. It takes time to grow young, even if one has had the
good fortune to escape or overcome the deformations of the
traditional socialization process. As we have seen in considering
the neotenous behavioral traits of the child, growing young is a
habit best acquired in childhood. Our conception of old age is a
bad habit to which most of us have been conditioned too early.
What may be called "statutory old age" is something of which
the child is soon made aware. In the Western world the child as
he develops learns to perceive "old age" as something quite
removed from himself, from the way he feels about himself.
"Really old people" are conceived as being out of their time,
anachronistic, parodies of something they once were. To be old,

in short, is to be contemptible. Such views were, of course, conditioned by the attitudes of the young prevailing in the Anglo-Saxon part of the Western world. The young condescend to the old, and demand that they conform to their expectations of them. In this manner the old come to suffer that ultimate denial of uniqueness and identity that is so uncomprehendingly and heartlessly imposed upon them. The segregation that exists between age groups in the Anglo-Saxon–speaking world creates an "agist" prejudice, akin to that of the "racist" for whom

> Through the distorting glass of Prejudice
> All nature seems awry, and but its own
> Wide-warped creations straight.

From such an agist viewpoint, aging is seen to be a biodegradable process, the inexorable progress of which leads to breakdown and the grave. Everyone in our culture is discouraged from accepting himself as he really is, but is expected to measure up or down to the age-grade role he is expected to play. Old people are expected to conform to the statutory requirements of old age. Violations of the rule are negatively sanctioned. At sixty or so one must retire from the job, which for many means retirement from life, to be completely out of the run of things, to be removed from positions of influence, to be "put out to pasture," to become a "Senior Citizen," a euphemism for superannuation, relegation to the periphery of the outskirts of society.

If our old are senescent it is for the most part our society, whose ideas on aging are senescent, that has made them so. We are a society that, because of its antiquated ideas on the nature of human growth and development, is severely weakening itself for want of new and youthful ideas. This is particularly true of a period in which social change is approaching an exponential rate. The attempts to solve new problems with old ideas simply will not work. Hence the importance of recognizing that unless we adjust ourselves to these changes in time we may go the way of the dodo, become obsolete as a society because we failed to recognize the value of paedomorphism and continued along the road of gerontomorphism.

We have grown old in our ways. We seem unable or unwilling to keep abreast of the knowledge that has already been acquired. With respect to our understanding of behavioral growth in a world grown gerontomorphic, in the sense that it has grown old in its outmoded ways, we are in the position of a centenarian attempting to run a mile race with a twenty-year-old Olympic competitor.

Too many among us have been waylaid by age and surprised by Time, ready to resign, to submit, to surrender to the myth of "old age." Most people seem convinced that since the body inevitably shows the "ravages" of Time, similar ravages must therefore affect the mind, the spirit. Not true. What is most important is that in our lives we have learned through the mind, the mind that is our spirit, and that is what will remain even when the body breaks down.

It is not with the prolongation of life that we should be so much concerned as with the prolongation of our paedomorphic drives, the prolongation of our youthfulness, the prolongation of the quality of life, the realization of our destiny. It is not so much the arrest or reversal of the physical processes of aging that should concern us, as the realization of potentialities for healthful behavioral and psychological growth, potentialities with which we are so generously endowed and which we have so little understood.

To grow young means to grow in our youthful traits, *not* to grow out of or to abandon them. The gospel of the Western world is that the object of growth is to become a "mature adult," to grow from childhood through adolescence to adulthood. The child is enjoined to "grow up," which means "upward" toward adulthood, and this becomes his ideal. Nothing can match his impatience to do so. He comes to identify "growing up" in height with "growing up" in adult stature. The conventional wisdom requires that all "childish" traits be left behind just as one does one's outworn clothes. The emphasis is pejorative. From their "mature adult" heights adults only too frequently look down patronizingly upon the "childish" qualities of the child, without any understanding of their real meaning. Such adults fail to understand that those "childish" qualities constitute the most valuable possessions of our species, to be cherished, nurtured, and cultivated. They fail to realize that the child surpasses the adult by the wealth of his possibilities. In a very real sense infants and children implicitly know a great deal more about many aspects of growing than do adults; adults, therefore, have more to learn from them about these matters than the latter have to learn from adults. Children have a world of their own for us to know.

From their "mature" heights, adults for the most part ignore the clear meaning of the child's neotenous traits and crassly perceive them as belonging to the same class of behavior as whining, self-centeredness, self-pity, obstinacy, impatience, impetuousness, practical joking, and the like. Indeed, these are behaviors often observed in children, but they are usually the product of poor socialization of which the children have been the victims. What we call "childish" behavior constitutes a reflection of the inadequacies of the socializers, and is in no way to be regarded as the expression of the child's natural drives. Equally certainly such behaviors have no relation whatever to the neotenous behavioral traits of children. It is, however, a common practice to attribute many behavioral traits, especially of children, to some innate, hereditary, or group cause. That "cause" is then given a label and the word becomes a "reality," such as "childishness," and since it has been given a name, "childishness" then becomes a proof of its existence.

It is very difficult for most people to break out of this kind of circular reasoning, which makes it all the more necessary that those of us who are able to rethink our ideas and prejudices in the light of the facts should do so. False ideas falsify the perception of reality. If the young subscribe to false ideas relating to the old, it is as nothing compared to the unsound ideas that adults hold and put into effect in relation to the young. Where the correction of those erroneous ideas should begin or, preferably, their avoidance, is in childhood. In healthy socialization, in which parents, teachers, and other socializers understand the requirements of the child for growth and development, the growing mutual respect and love render obsolete the traditional prejudices and obviate the tyranny that adults customarily exercise over children.

Children are the tools who, when we allow them to, help us to sculpt, as it were, our way toward humanity; in bringing them up we face ourselves, as in a mirror, in a clearer, brighter light.

Adults, while acknowledging—it would sometimes seem reluctantly—that children are human, only too often regard them as if they were intruders, or as something resembling raw materials, which it is their lot to fashion into the finished article, namely, faithful replicas of themselves. But children are neither intruders nor raw materials. They are highly organized creatures, with inbuilt behavioral drives directed toward continued growth and development. What they require for that continued growth and development is the recognition of the meaning of their neotenous drives and the expected appropriate satisfactions, stimulations, and encouragements.

Our culture requires that children must "grow up" to become adults and, since every child is taught that this is his chief goal in life, he grows to accept this belief unquestioningly. Success for the child becomes emulation of his elders. The rare individuals who somehow manage to avoid falling into this trap and retain their childlike qualities are considered either eccentric, odd, nonconformist, or otherwise otiose. We do not appreciate nonconformists in America. Our colleges and universities, not to mention our schools, avoid or reject them. A kind of ritual admiration exists for individuality, but it is neither cherished nor encouraged. In England, by contrast, individuality, eccentricity, are both admired and prized. No one has put the case for the nonconformist and the eccentric better than John Stuart Mill (1806–1873), when he wrote in 1859, in that peerless tract *On Liberty*,

> The mere example of non-conformity, the mere refusal to bend the knee to custom, is itself a service. Precisely because the tyranny of opinion is such as to make eccentricity a reproach, it is desirable to break through that tyranny, that people should be eccentric. Eccentricity has always abounded where strength of character has abounded, and the amount of eccentricity in a society has generally been proportional to the amount of genius, vigour, and moral courage which it contained. That so few now dare to be eccentric, marks the chief danger of the time.

It is a danger that has increased with time. Nonconformity is regarded as itself dangerous; as something to be feared and even punished, for nonconformists have a way of questioning our most fundamental and cherished beliefs. They tend to see things in an unhabitual way. They rock the boat and make one feel both uncomfortable and unhappy. To the self-serving flagwavers who have redefined patriotism to serve their own ends they are subversive and unpatriotic. And yet, in spite of the antipathy toward them, eccentrics, like cheerfulness, will keep creeping in to challenge the complacent and the orthodox. They are usually uninstitutionalized academically—that is to say, academically unacceptable—so they work outside institutional settings as independent spirits; like so many candles they cast light all around them, only too often at the cost of their own consumption.

We sometimes speak of "the childlike quality of genius," or we say of an especially gifted person's way of looking at things that "it is the child in him." William Cowper (1731–1800) spoke of Isaac Newton as the "childlike sage! Sagacious reader of the words of God." Someone, with deep insight, has said that genius is the recovery of childhood at will. That's pretty good, but what is better is that the genius of the child could be realized for every human in a society that applied the understanding of neoteny to the rearing of children. Such humans would be realized and fulfilled beings compared to what adults for the most part are today: deteriorated children. Our goal, so seldom realized, should be directed not merely toward the realization of the optimum development of the unique potentialities with which each child is born, but also toward the full realization of the child's neotenous traits. We should not then have to worry much about "growing older," or "old age," since, having grown young, the only problems of chronologic aging with which we would have to contend would be those of illness, disorder, or disease, as well as those infirmities that will certainly strike some individuals as a consequence of breakdown in some organ or system.

It cannot be too often repeated that the growing old of the body does not mean that the spirit has to grow old too. The point I wish most strongly to emphasize here is that every bit of relevant evidence indicates that infirmities and breakdowns are much less likely to occur in those who have retained a youthful spirit than in those who have succumbed to the self-fulfilling prophecy of aging, and have aged in accordance with what is ritually expected of them. The whole of psychosomatic and holistic medicine testifies to that fact. Age, as someone has said, is where you're at in your head, an attitude of mind.

The Mythology of Aging

The mythology of aging from the alleged "childishness" of the child to "the second childhood" of the adult paints a picture of progressively inevitable breakdown and decrepitude, mental and physical, which is very destructive indeed.

> And what's a life?—a weary pilgrimage,
> Whose glory in one day doth fill the stage
> With childhood, manhood, and decrepit age.

When Francis Quarles (1592–1644) wrote these lines in 1635, the average duration of life of Europeans was 33⅓ years. The average duration of life has today risen to more than twice that, and it has been done not so much by medicine, not by drugs, and not by anything other than the application of sound thinking to the improvement of the conditions of daily living. What has been achieved for the extension of the *duration* of life by sound thinking can also be achieved by the same means for the improvement of the *quality* of life.

It has been true and continues to be true that

> Crabbed age and youth cannot live together:
>   Youth is full of pleasance, age is full of care;
> Youth like summer morn, age like winter weather;
>   Youth like summer brave, age like winter bare.
> Youth is full of sport, age's breath is short;
>   Youth is nimble, age is lame;
> Youth is hot and bold, age is weak and cold;
>   Youth is wild, and age is tame.
> Age, I do abhor thee; youth, I do adore thee;
>   O, my love, my love is young!
> Age, I do defy thee: O, sweet shepherd, hie thee,
>   For methinks thou stay'st too long.
>
> SHAKESPEARE
> *The Passionate Pilgrim*

Indeed, there has been a further erosion of rapport between the young and old since those lines were written. But it need not be so, for age does not have to be either crabbed or full of care. That is an antique idea that belongs to the past. To the future belongs the notion that age is a period when the consolidated experience of life has grown into that wisdom of the long-distance runner who has husbanded his resources in such a manner that he completes the course with energy to spare. Far from being crabbed, the older person will be expected to continue in the neotenous optimistic frame of mind with which he commenced. Just as one learns to be crabbed and full of care, one can learn to be cheerful, optimistic, full of laughter, and caring for others.

Among the most pervasive of the myths relating to aging is the canard of "second childhood." Aristophanes (c. 450–385 B.C.), in his play *Clouds,* notes that "Old men are children for a second time" (1417). In *Hamlet,* Rosencrantz says, "They say an old man is twice a child." Yes, "they say," but it is not true. All of us have known men and women who remained youthful all the days of their lives, well into their eighties and even later. The great sense of fun and joyfulness of Einstein, his remarkable youthfulness, has seldom been commented on, but was very evident to all who knew him. Bertrand Russell was another outstanding example of a man who retained his youthfulness into the nineties, and so did Erich Kahler, who was an outstanding example of a man who had grown in all his neotenous qualities almost to perfection, who remained hale and hearty up to the last weeks of his life, when cancer finally extinguished him. These men were hard at work, with minds as clear as they had ever been, when death overtook them. The uniqueness of each human makes a tragedy of death, and during our sojourn on earth death hangs over us all like a kind of invisible darkness in the sunlight. But while we live it is the sunlight that warms us, and we must know that the sun will continue to shine upon us while we live with the reality of death by filling the void with the permanence of fulfillment and achievement, the fulfillment and achievement of being human.

Probably the most delightful example of young-spiritedness in old age is Eubie Blake, composer and jazz pianist who at 97 is still composing and giving concerts. Among women in their eighties and nineties outstanding examples of young-spiritedness are the actresses Gladys Cooper now, alas, no longer with us, and Eva Le Gallienne and Cathleen Nesbitt, both still delighting audiences, Martha Graham, dancer and choreographer, and the English writers Florida Scott-Maxwell, Rebecca West, and Doris Langley Moore, not to mention many others.

Of course, all of us have known men and women who have prematurely aged, who have broken down either physically or mentally or both, at what seemed to us an earlier age than one would have expected. At their age they should have been much younger. Most of us have also known old men and women who have deteriorated either mentally or physically or both. But has that ever seemed "natural" to any of us? In some cases, perhaps, but many such old people I have known have seemed to me in a condition that could have been somehow either wholly or partly avoided or mitigated, "if only they had lived right," if only they had lived neotenously. In her inspiring book, *Your Second Life,* Gay Luce tells the story of the organization she founded called Senior Actualization and Growth Explorations (SAGE), of the great changes brought about in those who had been abandoned to old age, the revitalization and re-creativity of their lives. She lists the stereotypes of our culture as saying that:

Old people should be dignified and circumspect
Old dogs can't learn new tricks
Old people are closed-minded, set in their ways, slow, senile
Old people are ugly
There is no future for old people. Why teach them?
Old people don't want to use or touch their bodies
Old people like to sit still and be quiet.

Gay Luce didn't believe these ideas had any validity, nor did her friends; so they decided to experiment. "If we created something like the situation in which children grow," she writes, "wouldn't we all grow?"

This was a stroke of genius, for intuitively or otherwise, Gay and her colleagues grasped the principle of growth through neoteny, and the disastrous effects of living up to other people's conventional expectations. "Out of ignorance," Dr. Luce writes, "about the basics of health we abuse and neglect ourselves for fifty or sixty years and then react with indignation, surprise, or grief when we find ourselves with intractable ailments, aches, stiffness, or arthritis. Life is movement. City dwelling is mostly sedentary. Look at the child, restless, tumbling upside down, expressing his feelings freely, and exploring himself." Dr. Luce points out what cannot be too often emphasized, namely, that limberness diminishes with reduced movement, and that ideas, feelings, playfulness also diminish with reduced expression. The diminished become quiet, withdrawn, unexpressive.

As Dr. Luce says, it is not the years themselves that diminish us. It is the way we have learned to live them, giving up a little of our true selves at each step. In our culture we lack a tradition of self-development for the elderly; what we have instead is a tradition of not-so-benign neglect and uselessness. This is supported by the established mythology relating to aging.

Myths are idealizations of social conditions; their main function is to satisfy the needs of the group. Myths are a people's way of perceiving the truth. Related to a fundamental reality of life such as aging and the aged, the real and the self-serving are fused into a way of perceiving things that becomes reality itself. Such myths are made to correspond to, and often to have the force of, biological and statutory laws. In this manner the myth is endowed with the aura of scientific, legalistic, and historical sanctity. As such, myths often assume an ideological power that becomes the basis for unsound attitudes and practices. The myths relating to aging resemble those of racism, and we all know to what atrocities and injustices such mythology has led. As Voltaire remarked, those who believe in absurdities will commit atrocities.

Among the most atrocious of these absurdities is the widespread belief, upon which we have already touched, that old age is a kind of "second childhood," with the word "childhood" used in a pejorative sense, the implication being that with age there is an inexorable deterioration of the mental faculties so that sophisticated adult traits are lost and there is a regression to the simpler traits of the child. This is utter nonsense. Aging, except in rare pathological instances, is not a regression to a childhood condition. There *are* such things as "presenile dementia" (Alzheimer's disease) and "senile dementia," which until very recently were thought to be an inevitable consequence of aging in many men and women. Presenile dementia has its onset in the forties, senile dementia in the sixties. They affect over a million Americans—that is, some 5 percent of the elderly population. The devastating deterioration of the mind represented by these dementias is so severe, incapacitating, and pathetic that once seen, the impression likely to be left is that this is what "old age," "senility," is really like. Nothing could be further from the truth. Five percent of 250 million is a sizable number of people. We now have hope of reducing that number to the vanishing point.

The accumulating evidence drawn from the newest researches on aging, in addition to destroying a good many myths about aging, more positively holds out promise of a future in which the physical and mental breakdown associated with old age will be greatly ameliorated or altogether eliminated. Were our government to spend as much money on research devoted to the processes of aging as it spends on a single moon shot that future could be brought very close to us all. As one of the leading researchers in the field, Dr. Bernard L. Strehler, said, "One reason that aging has not received the emphasis it deserves has to do with the aging of bureaucracies themselves. New bureaus and institutes are often vital organizations; as they grow older they are concerned more with maintaining the status quo than with imaginative progress."

After much politicizing a National Institute on Aging was established in 1974 as an agency of the National Institutes of Health, empowered to conduct and support "biomedical, social, and behavioral research and training related to the aging process and the diseases and other special problems and needs of the aged."

The understanding and the control of the aging process is within our grasp. As a first step all that is required is greater financial support than is at present being made available for research in this area. Assuming an intensive attack on the problems of aging, it is agreed by most experts that within ten years we could understand in depth the details of cellular and bodily aging and, probably, how to control that process. Let me here quote Dr. Strehler once more:

> The eventual understanding and control of the aging process will cause a revolution in human affairs. Already a few studies are under way on the social consequences of greatly retarding or abolishing aging and death. A few misconceptions should, however, first be laid to rest. Some of the evidently misinformed opponents of greater, healthy life-spans seem to believe that the world would become populated with decrepit, patched-up, wizened, senile people, perhaps fed through tubes and moving with the aid of electronic prostheses. This ugly picture is totally false, for there is no way to appreciably increase life-span except by improving the body's physical state. Instead, humans that live for 150 years or more will be healthy for a much greater percentage of their total life-span. Men and women of highly advanced age will possess bodies like those of much younger people. In fact, their minds will be even more improved, for the greater years of optimum health will provide more opportunity to assimilate the world's wonders and lead to a greater measure of wisdom—the only intellectual commodity that often improves with age.

There are many other beneficial individual and social changes that will ensue under this new dispensation. The future will see a doubling of the healthy middle years from the present thirty or forty years. Middle age will be greatly extended, as will all other developmental periods. The consequences of this alone will be revolutionary, for it will mean that in virtually all areas of creative and productive life the human experience will be greatly enlarged. Each of us will not only know more, but our ability to integrate what we at present regard as different branches of knowledge will be greatly increased. The age of specialization will make way for the Age of Integration, for interdisciplinary thinking and research, and an altogether wider and deeper appreciation of the world in which we live and of our fellow creatures. The improvement in the conditions of aging will represent but the realization of the inbuilt requirements of the later stages of growth and development, not as a final affliction, but as a happy fulfillment.

If we add to all this neotenous growth and development the purely social achievements that will accompany it, the world will be a much pleasanter place for everyone to live in.

Historically, aging has been viewed as an affliction or an abnormal departure from health. As Seneca (c. 4 B.C.–65 A.D.), the Roman philosopher, stated that view two thousand years ago, "Old age is a sickness from which one never recovers." Through the centuries that has been the conclusion of most older people who have delivered themselves on the subject. This has been especially true in a society such as ours, in which old age is treated as if it were an offense that carried its own penalty.

Too many people become shipwrecked by old age simply because they have never learned how to navigate the waters in which they suddenly find themselves. They find themselves in unfamiliar territory, traumatically displaced persons consigned to the very outskirts of the society of which they were once full members, forced into a lifestyle for which they have not been prepared, a lifestyle of unstructured time and reduced input from the world with which they were once familiar. The feeling is one of abandonment, of lack of caring by that world, a kind of exile or excommunication.

One should always bear in mind that most older people do not become bedridden, but all of us need to be cared for, for caring—the other word for love—is what we need all the days of our lives, not only to be cared for, but also to care for others. Who was it who said that the real vocation of the old is to give out love?

Children love the old; they seem to have a special affinity for them, and where experiments have been conducted in bringing children into association with the old in institutions, the most beneficial changes have been brought about in the condition of the residents. Grandparents often seem to enjoy their grandchildren rather more than the parents do. Here is a wide-open field ready for further exploration.

The old are a biological élite, for they have withstood the assaults and insults upon their integrity that have caused the demise of the less vigorous. The old have used their biological resources well.

Assaults and Insults of the Environment

Among the principal assaults and insults of the environment upon the aging are the drugs prescribed by the medical profession, presumably to meet the problems of the aged with which they, as a profession, are confronted. The average American sixty-five or older takes thirteen different drugs a year. Since, with aging, changes occur in liver and kidney functions that affect the processes of metabolism, this often means that symptoms attributed to senility are in fact due to dangerous chemical mixes. Among other things the elderly have a lower oxygen pressure than the young and are therefore particularly vulnerable to deficient blood oxygenation, which can be induced by many drugs, such as sleeping pills. In this connection it should be noted that among the most influential contributors to the mythology of aging are physicians. Dr. Robert Butler, Director of the National Institute of Aging and Pulitzer Prize-winning author of *Why Survive? Growing Old in America,* speaking at the annual meeting of the American Psychiatric Association in 1978, commented that the thought of treating older patients unnerves thousands of American physicians, who consider themselves successful only when they "cure" patients. Many physicians, he noted, feel frustrated because they are unable to meet the needs of the older patient.

Other reasons for physician frustration with elderly patients are that the aged are "near death anyway," personal fears about old age, and personal conflicts about relationships with parental figures that may be aroused by contacts with elderly patients. Dr. Butler urged on physicians the necessity of overcoming the ambivalence, negativism, and the sense of threat that the realities of aging will increasingly present.

Since today older patients account for some 40 percent of the physician's office time and some 30 percent of his hospital time, the training and attitudes of physicians in meeting the needs of the elderly call for a radical change. This is especially necessary in view of the demographic revolution ahead of us: During the first quarter of the next century one out of five Americans will be over sixty-five, and physicians may be spending at least 75 percent of their time with older patients. Like it or not, all physicians will have to become geriatricians.

When professionals and laymen alike believe that nothing can be done for the elderly who "inevitably" are in poor condition, the stage is set for the aged to feel frustration, hostility, paranoia, depression, abandonment, and indifference toward others. Hence the stereotype of the cantankerous, sullen, apathetic, or unresponsive older person is more likely to become a reality. Action and reaction tend to perpetuate what is essentially a quagmire of confused and unsound thinking leading to equally confused and unsound conduct—the mythology of aging. Under such conditions the aged are forced into a purposeless existence and a self-indulgent mindlessness, falling out of all consideration and becoming victims of the ultimate dread of becoming a "cabbage." Such attitudes will surely become a thing of the past in what Ronald Blythe has called "the sprawling new commonwealth of the aged," for what we believe to be "old age" today will be something very much more agreeable tomorrow.

Mental Abilities

The notion that ability and achievement are at their maximum in the early years and then decline as one ages originated in a period when the majority of people enjoyed rather shorter life-spans than most people do today. The truth is that the peak of creativity remains high in later years, as witnessed by such men as Leonardo da Vinci, Michelangelo, Victor Hugo, Tennyson, Thomas Hardy, Alexander Graham Bell, Verdi, Lizst, Benjamin Franklin, Thomas Jefferson, Bertrand Russell, and innumerable others. Verdi was eighty-five when he composed *Te Deum;* Tennyson was eighty when he wrote "Crossing the Bar"; Eubie Blake at ninety-seven, jazz pianist and composer, is still playing and composing. Alberta Hunter, at eighty-six, is still delighting audiences with her singing, and in May 1981 received the second annual Tribute to Black Women Award for her lifelong contributions to black music and an "inner spirit" that, the award said, "glides along on wings of jazz and blues."

Michelangelo was eighty-nine when he painted some of his greatest masterpieces; Viscount Bryce, author of *The American*

Commonwealth, was over eighty when he wrote his great work, *Modern Democracies.* It was said of him that whenever he happens to die, he will die young.

It was William Hazlitt (1778–1830), English essayist and critic, who remarked that "the worst of old age is that of the mind." It is a view of old age that has for too long prevailed. Recent research has thoroughly discredited the myth of the inevitability of mental deterioration with age. The fact is that there is a great deal of variability in the processes of aging, and their effects are by no means uniform. Some attributes become weaker with age, others stronger. Memory may decline, but understanding usually improves.

In many older people there is a clear slowing-down of mental alertness, in information processing. Stored knowledge may increase, but the search for it, and its retrieval, may be slower than it used to be. This should not be regarded as a disability or as evidence of mental decline. As Dr. James E. Birren, Director of the University of Southern California's Ethel and Percy Andrus Gerontology Center, has said,

> With maturation comes a great conceptual grasp so that we can size up the situation and then look to the relevant items in our store. This is what I call the race between the chunks and the bits. While younger people, say those between eighteen and twenty-two, can process more bits per second, and even though by age sixty, that number may be halved, the older person may process bigger chunks. The race may go to the tortoise because he is chunking, and not to the hare because he is just bitting along.

It may be that you can't teach an old dog new tricks, but that is certainly not so in the case of older people. There is much evidence, both experimental and observational, that far from decreasing with age, both learning ability and IQ remain steady, and in many cases even increase. IQ tests should not be confused with the power and the ability of the intellect to function. As Dr. G. Haydu has put it, "the intellect is the capacity to see, and manage, apply, combine, and recombine what the individual finds meaningful and significant in his world, which of course is his cultural world. This capacity does not suffer decline, except in terminal senescence.''

Experimental and other studies in recent years on the relation between aging and brain and behavior have revealed that there is a progressive decline in postmaturational brain cell efficiency. Functionally, this decline in brain cell efficiency is expressed in cellular information loss, that is, in cell information content, but not necessarily in information-processing and analysis. The latter processes may slow down in the aged, but they work just as unerringly as in the young—especially among those older persons who have led continuously active lives, who have not allowed their minds to harden into conservatism from, among other things, lack of exercise. Many early studies on aging were done on general or mental hospital patients, and the findings on these desperate people somehow were generalized to the aged as a whole. Professor Marian Diamond of the University of California at Berkeley has recently surveyed the evidence with particular reference to cellular changes in the human brain in the aging, and also in the aging rat brain, and has concluded that ''in the absence of disease, impoverished environment, or poor nutrition, the nervous system apparently does have the potential to oppose marked deterioration with aging.'' The truth seems to be that there is extensive neuronal loss during the development of the nervous system in young animals, after which the brain cell number remains remarkably constant. This was the conclusion already arrived at many years ago by C. S. Minot, distinguished Johns Hopkins anatomist, in his book *The Problem of Age, Growth, and Death,* published in 1908. What he wrote then has been abundantly confirmed since: ''The period of old age, so far from being the chief period of decline, is in reality essentially the period in which the actual decline going on in each of us will be least''; to this the contemporary anatomist Professor Diamond adds, ''This is especially true as long as the brain is exposed to a stimulating environment.'' And a stimulating environment is one that we can always make for ourselves, if ever and whenever the external world fails to provide it. It takes effort to keep young.

Functional or social deterioration in the aging has often been confused with brain deterioration. This is an error. Depression, when it occurs, is often accompanied by psychomotor retardation, disorientation, feelings of apathy, hostility, low self-esteem, low attention span, loss of sense of humor, loss of libido, and general helplessness. In institutions the aged are often likely to suffer from loneliness and sensory deprivation, which may worsen existing problems and may intensify or even create depression. It is now well established that the elderly who remain in the home environment or have the company of a spouse for a long time show a much lower incidence of brain or social deterioration.

Money is frequently a problem. But a well-organized society, one genuinely concerned for the welfare of its elder citizens, could easily take care of that. Professor David Hackett Fischer of Brandeis University has proposed a plan that is simplicity itself. Let me give it in his own words.

Instead of supporting elderly people by grants of income at the end of life, it would be cheaper, easier, and less disagreeable in many ways to give each American a grant of capital at the beginning of life instead. Small capital payments would be more effective than large payments in the form of income.

Many American banks offer seven-year savings certificates which pay an interest of 9 percent a year. It is doubtful whether interest rates will remain that high, but given the record of the Federal Reserve Board they are not likely to fall very far. Let us assume that on long-term investments, interest of 8 percent will be generally available. Suppose that every American received at birth a sort of "national inheritance"—a gift of capital in the amount of $1,400. The gift would be surrounded with many restrictions. It could never be spent, loaned, borrowed, alienated, expended, or employed as collateral in any way. This capital sum would be invested—perhaps in a savings account, or in government securities. The money would not be taxable. It would be left to earn compound interest until the infant who originally received it reached the age of sixty-five. At 8 percent, over sixty-five years, the original $1,400 would grow to $225,000!

At the age of sixty-five, the income from $225,000 would provide an old-age pension. At 7 percent the pension would be more than $15,000 for each American—far more than Social Security provides today. A husband and wife together would have a nontaxable house-

hold income of more than $31,000 a year. Upon their death, the
money would return to the Treasury.

Yet the cost to the public would consist only of the initial payment
of the original capital sum to each American child.

As Professor Fischer goes on to show, the cost of such an arrangement would be $4.2 billion—a small fraction of present
expenditure for social insurance. In 1974 alone the American
government spent roughly $100 billion for that purpose—nearly
$60 billion for Social Security alone.

With age, biochemical changes occur in the brain, usually in
the form of depletion of various enzymes and other substances,
and some differential cell loss in the gray matter of the cerebrum
(large brain), cerebellum (little brain), and brain stem. Loss of
cells in the cerebellum and brain stem may account for the loss
of locomotor stability in some elderly people. No one has ever
counted the cells at different ages over the whole of the gray
matter. It may well be that cell loss occurs at different rates
in different areas of the gray matter; we have some evidence
for this in the work of Brody, who counted the cortical cells
in seven areas of the brain. Brody's findings are shown in
Table VII.

Brody found that from birth until eighteen years of age, packing density in some areas fell by 61 to 78 percent, while in other
areas the decrease was less, from 40 to 52 percent. Between
eighteen and forty-five years the packing density falls sharply,
and continues to fall until ninety-five years of age. It will be
observed from Table VII that there is appreciable variability in
the number of cells present at each of the four ages, and that
there is not a very considerable loss of cells between the ages of
forty-five and ninety-five; in some areas of the brain there actually appeared to be a greater number of cells present at ninety-
five than there were at forty-five years of age.

It is sometimes stated in articles and books on the brain that
from the age of twenty-five years onward one loses between
50,000 and 100,000 cortical cells a day, which would make the
loss between 2,000 and 4,000 an hour. The reader should not be
alarmed, for several reasons: first, because there has been no
really adequate investigation of the daily or even yearly loss of

TABLE VII

Relation of Cell Number in Cortical Sections with Age

Specimen—Age	D	G	I	L
HC 3—Newborn	3706	2222	4576	2838
HC 6— 1 day	2644		3072	2843
HC 7— 2 days	3430		4294	3253
HC 21— 2 months	2653	2874	2890	2835
HC 13—16 years	1530	1512	2187	2648
HC 1—18 years	1317	1338	2072	2565
HC 11—18 years	1385	1488		2570
HC 2—19 years	1460	1396	2106	2596
HC 18—21 years	1701	1503		2448
HC 10—45 years	1399	1126		1740
HC 19—48 years	1215	1176	1950	1916
HC 17—70 years			1271	1243
HC 9—73 years	996	1332	1194	1837
HC 16—74 years	1009	1595	1165	
HC 8—75 years	994	1375	1092	1800
HC 12—75 years	977		1063	1802
HC 20—78 years	1206	1241	1055	1840
HC 4—80 years	886	1932	970	1810
HC 15—81 years	1016		991	1489
HC 5—95 years	910	1763	887	1773

D, Precentral gyrus; G, Postcentral gyrus; L, Area striata,
I Superior temporal gyrus (After Brody)

brain cells; second, because at birth we are endowed with about 16 billion cells or neurons in the cortex alone, so that by the age of seventy we would still have some 15 billion left; and third, even if it were true that we lost 100,000 neurons a day, let us say about 10 percent between the ages of twenty and seventy, that does not mean that we would necessarily be 10 percent less efficient, because the great superfluity (redundancy) of neurons always present in the brain, and the many possible additional connections they are capable of establishing with other neurons, allows for the loss of great quantities of them without significant loss of brain complexity and power.

Current investigations suggest that while some cell loss may occur with age it will vary in different individuals and will occur at different rates in the areas and parts of the brain affected. But such losses, as we have already remarked, can be compensated for by an active mind and a stimulating environment. An active mind can be self-stimulating and thus always create its own environment. A stimulating external environment can induce activity in a brain that might otherwise remain sluggish. Atrophy from disuse is most likely to occur in a brain that is inadequately stimulated, whether the stimulation is from within or without. The best thing is to enjoy the advantages of both kinds of stimulation, those that draw upon past experience and those that are novel and challenging, a combination that continuously enriches the lives of those who grow young. New ideas, like new experiences, are the lifeblood of the mind. Old age constitutes no barrier to that kind of continuing excitement. The brain is a very receptive and lively organ, which thrives on activity, accounting for as much as 10 percent of the total expenditure of energy and 25 percent of the total oxygen consumption of the whole body. This enormous expenditure of energy by brain cells means that an extraordinary amount of metabolic activity continually takes place in the brain and its appendages. That energy is there for use, as are the superabundant brain cells. It has been claimed that we use only about 10 percent of our brain cells. I have not been able to trace the source of that claim, but it may well be an understatement.

It has also been stated that each of the 16 billion neurons in the cortex is capable of establishing connections with from 25,000 to 75,000 or more other neurons. This is achieved by the growth of collaterals from the neurons. It has long been established that neuronal collaterals actively grow in response to externally stimulating environments. It has further been established that impoverished environments have the effect of reducing the growth of collaterals, and result in reduced brain size. It has been thought that when this occurs in infancy and childhood, the damage done to the brain is irreversible. Investigation, happily, has shown that this is not the case and that the growth potentials of the brain are such that with improved conditions the "damage" is reversible. The so-called "damage" done to the brain that has suffered from an impoverished environment is qualitative, not quantitative. Stimulating environments produce more activity and more interaction with ideas and other people. The other people respond, and in so doing create a new dimension of interaction at a higher level of stimulation. This makes for better brain functioning and a more developed mind. So let there be no more talk of the brains we have lost, and more talk of what we can do with the brains that we have.

For most older people, the "difficulty" is not that they feel old, but that they don't. Florida Scott-Maxwell, the gifted English writer, when in her eighties, spoke of this feeling as an aspect of age

> almost embarrassing to speak of because of its extreme improbability. One wants to shield it from younger ears. Yet it is innocent, and may be forgiven us. It is this—the old feel very young. At moments, that is. Though we are aching, inadequate wrecks, there are times when, in our hearts, we are incurably, deliciously young. I have no idea whether we should or we should not be. Who is to say? Undoubtedly the quality of this strange youthfulness matters greatly. And observation tells us that it varies greatly. All that I am sure of is that an unexpected freshness comes to one when one is old. . . . This puzzling newness is so buoyant a thing it is a problem how to deal with it discreetly. Explain it as you will, it feels like happiness: but also release and exemption. . . . It must be honoured greatly, for the leap of expectancy that rises in its heart is authentic, and I beg you to believe me when I say it is pristine in its freshness.

It is interesting that in his book *The View in Winter: Reflections on Old Age,* Ronald Blythe found many of the English villagers of all classes whom he interviewed saying the same thing, and also commenting on the particular happiness that belonged to old age. All of which strongly supports the idea that the image we have of ourselves, relating both to our appearance and the way we feel about ourselves, probably represents a neotenous trait, a trait that has hardly been recognized, and certainly not understood. What it means is that we, all of us, carry within ourselves the core, the essence, of an eternally youthful spirit whose inner light is designed to warm and illuminate all the days of our lives. It is the unconquerable you, the you that cries out to be honored, and though overlaid by centuries of folly, continues to endure, and hence is recoverable at will. Do not let others impose upon you the mythology of "old age," for to feel young, even in many cases invigorated, is natural. It is a paedomorphic trait, which should reach its fullest expression in the later years, for what is "old age" designed to be if not the fulfillment of childhood promises, the fullest expression of childhood, of youthfulness?

I have shown that deterioration of the brain, except in a small proportion of cases, is not a necessary accompaniment of aging, and that for most of us the brain is capable of continuing to function in old age at a high level of efficiency, if it is continually exercised. There exists, therefore, no barrier in the later years to continued productivity and the enjoyment of new experiences, to creativity. We grow toward light, not toward darkness. The elderly have been lulled into the belief and forced into a position in which little or no effort is required of them; it is for that reason that so many of them become apathetic and fade away, wondering how they became such functionless effigies. Therefore, *never* retire. As Alex Comfort has remarked, a good retirement should last about two weeks. Older people need a sustained sense of achievement through work perhaps even more than younger people do. Mandatory retirement at an increasingly earlier age represents the self-destructive impulse of a myopic society.

The whole of life is a journey toward youthful old age, toward self-contemplation, love, gaiety, and, in a fundamental sense, the most gratifying time of our lives. Old age, like time, is a gift.

Until those past sixty become a political force they will continue to be treated as the untouchables of our society, and most of their real problems will continue to be overlooked. As a first step in the desired direction, what is needed is an organization akin to the Veterans of Foreign Wars, for most elderly people have been through in many ways more difficult and enduring conflicts than those who have fought in foreign wars. And as a second step, healthy people of middle age and younger should be placed in nursing homes in order to relearn how to become human beings. They might then emerge with some understanding of who it is that makes people feel old. In our assembly-line culture people become obsolete before their time. We no longer grow old gracefully. Years of experience are slighted and passed over. Instead of utilizing the accumulated experience and wisdom of the old to help solve our problems, we have turned the aged themselves into a problem. Our preoccupation with youth has made us forget that people considered "too old" often have the youngest ideas of all. "Old age" should be a harvest time when the riches of life are reaped and enjoyed, while it continues to be a special period for self-development and expansion, instead of a half-life waiting to die. And as for that, one needs a special strength to die, rather than a special weakness, and that strength can only come to us dying young, at whatever age that may be, neither surprised by time nor attenuated by it.

The old are able to enjoy life more than the young because they have a deeper understanding of it, because they are wiser. The old, indeed, are persons of especial worth, and in many societies are so regarded. The Chinese, for example, believe that a family that has an old person in it has a precious jewel.

In some older individuals, "where wasteful Time debateth with decay," the premises will break down long before the spirit is ready to vacate them. Yet all the evidence indicates that the principal factor in staving off the aging of the premises is youthfulness of spirit. This is why it is of the greatest urgency for contemporary humanity to understand the importance of the never-ending cultivation of the neotenous traits of the child, the continuous growth and development of those traits throughout life. In short, we must understand that we are designed to grow as children, *not* as what we misconceive adults to be.

Human worth is based on respect for the person, on the individual's inclusion in a community, on concern for the body, and on physical and spiritual needs. We are not alone in the world. The most pressing of all our drives is toward sociality, to be together with our friends, our fellow human beings. Sociality means involvement, interaction with others; and for this we must always make ourselves responsible. To be free to do as we please, we must be responsible for what we are pleased to do. The sense of responsibility does not develop without nurture; nurtured while young and exercised then, it becomes not a burden but a pleasure, for it is what we are pleased to do.

7

Import

In the preceding pages I have discussed the concept of neoteny
or paedomorphosis and the role it has played in the evolution of
humankind, not only physically but also behaviorally. In the
course of evolution these two modalities have proceeded interac-
tively and interrelatedly. The development of a large and complex brain, for example, made possible the large and more complex behavior of which humans alone are capable; this, in itself,
has led to all sorts of consequences, both behavioral and physical. We have seen that physical changes in form have been
brought about by the retention of fetal or juvenile traits, by the
slowing-down ("retardation") and extension of development.
What, however, has most interested us in this book has been not
so much the physical as the behavioral paedomorphism of humans and its consequences for human development. The discussion of the neotenic physical evolution of humanity, interesting
and important as it is, has mainly served to provide the scientific
underpinning for the application of the principle to the elucida-
tion of the role it has played in the evolution of human behavior.

What the reader will, I hope, have perceived is the central role
that neoteny has played in the evolution of our species, that

218

neoteny is the foundation source of our humanity, the great layer of flexibility that extends through the full duration of human life, from infancy through old age. I hope I have shown that what is required to maintain us as human, and to advance the depth and breadth of our humanity, is the favorable development of our neotenous traits.

What I have set before the reader in these pages will, I trust, be seen as a contribution to a new and more accurate vision of humankind, a vision that has the power to release the inner splendor in each of us.

It is on our new understanding of the real nature of humankind that we must take our stand, and it is especially here that we must redefine the nature of society. We must reject the notion of society as the institution that invents and creates enemies, and impounds all natural and human resources into its kneejerk terror, a society that is a machine solely for the generation of book values in the games played with human necessities.

Based on the evolutionary facts, we may define society as the nurturing life-system that generates and extends the neotenous traits of humanity with every generation. The perspective of evolution shows us that our neotenous, extended childhood, our lifelong youthfulness, becomes the single most commanding fact upon which to design all social and productive relations. The child, as Simone de Beauvoir has so well said, surpasses the adult by the wealth of his possibilities, the vast range of his acquisitions, and his emotional freshness. Throughout human history neotenic processes were sustained and succeeded within the evolutionary matrix because social organization rapidly evolved to support the demands of prolonged childhood, to afford the protection, nurturing, learning, and interpersonal support and collaboration essential to the continuing development of human potentialities.

The import of *Growing Young* constitutes no less than an open demand of our school systems that they be consciously and deliberately redesigned to serve the developmental aims and purposes latent and accessible in our children. Teaching itself must be reconceived, as essentially the discovery and revelation of order, rather than its futile, barren imposition. Process, context, and function must become the methodological interactive units of learning. *Performance* of every sort—from recitation to demonstration before the community—must be expected of each student, study group, and class. Acquiring skills and learning must be assured the student, whose confidence in his teachers and whose feelings of satisfaction in accomplishment will make the whole process of learning gratifying, and school itself both the earnest application of a lifetime and an era when he learned that learning is fun.

The problem that confronts us in this period of social disorganization and worn-out educational theory, beleaguered principals, terrified teachers, decayed and censored textbooks, and poverty-stricken pupils is not insuperable. We are the problem-solving species. It is quite within the power of intelligent, level-headed committees of parents and citizens in any community to develop policies of enlightened and enlivening schooling, then to involve special interests by appealing to their own personal self-interests in order to reach consensus, and finally to obtain the financial and local governmental support necessary to carry the programs through.

Our "primitive" forebears managed to teach each generation of children everything essential to a functionally independent life in the family or tribe's territory. They had names for every plant, knew the traits and habits of every animal, knew weaver's knots, flaking procedures, fire-making methods, shelter-building techniques, and the homely principles of first aid as well as relief for sickness. They knew the history of their people, could sing and recite the poems and the legends of their gods and heroes. They created their own religious systems as well as their own theories of knowledge and value, esthetics, morals, and metaphysics—all of them providing a feeling that made sense and order out of life, natural events, and the fate of the individual. This was directly consequential education. It worked as it was learned, as offering the development of knowledge and skills essential to survival.

Today education has lost its bearing in how to present itself as consequential. But the living pressure of the learning times of childhood—the time-phased opportunities of the developmental stages of childhood—compel attention, for the child is as much a part of life at five as at twenty-one, in his own terms and certainly in the terms of society.

Some years ago a friend of mine, Preston Tuttle, was asked to design an ideal school that would offer educational service to children from nursery school, about age two, through high school, about age eighteen. He set about this lovely task with a full spirit, bent upon a fully integrated enterprise in which the experiences of each age group would be shared with other age groups, and in which the older children would be expected to be active in teaching or tutoring the younger ones. The driving technique he counted on was the principle of *performance,* which was to transform the student body into a mutually shared learning community, in which each child supportively established an individual identity, the full features of which are quite clearly developed by age nine-and-a-half, like the face of a butterfly pupa, with firmer definition at adolescence, when the chitinous shell splits down the back and a wet-winged plumpish body emerges. Well, my friend's ideal school was nothing so much as a college—an assemblage of scholars and advanced-degree teachers where those graduating could expect to leave with qualifications for junior year entrance to any university in the land. As for personal development, especially in psychological strength and self-confidence, my friend feels it would have expunged neurosis, prepared each child to handle difficult persons, especially parents, and it would have turned out as graduates the most employable and socially the most honest and delightful personalities, and psychologically the most healthy to be found anywhere. His school, alas, was never established. Yet it remains a mandatory vision. Its authenticity resides in its tribal and primitive community character, which he more or less unconsciously followed in designing it. But if it had been built, he tells me, he thinks he would have to rename the main building today Neoteny Hall.

In the light of the facts it is clear that the main task of education should be the art and science of assisting the child to fulfill his promises. The child, so full of potentialities already awakened, is striving toward their realization at his own particular pace. The world, however, in which the child has lived so long is not accommodative to that pace. Most parents have wanted to get their children out of childhood as soon as possible. Whatever the reasons for their behavior, there is a massive failure to understand the importance of allowing children to proceed at their own rates of development, neither to retard nor to accelerate them.

The fact that the human baby has completed only half its gestation when it is born, and only brings it to a close when it begins to crawl about under its own steam at about ten months of age, means that during that period it is in an immature state. More than any other infant primate, the human requires a great deal of tender loving care. The infant is much more delicately poised in relation to the human environment than we have hitherto realized, and we need, therefore, to revise many of our approaches to that wonder of the world.

Babies are new to themselves, and all that surrounds them is novel. Children of all ages feel much the same way; it is a feeling and a view of life that can last a lifetime. To see the world always with a fresh eye means that one brings to every experience a habit of feeling, of experiencing, a not-taking-for-granted the everyday scene, but finding something new in it each time one encounters it. And this can only come about naturally by encouraging the child, at every age, to be interested, curious, and experimental-minded. This is what babies and children are, and what all humans are capable of being all of their lives, if only they receive the appropriate encouragements. Childhood remains the unforgotten world of enchantment, a rich treasury of a remembered world that touches experience at many points and enlivens it. In a world, however, in which children without childhood suffer from a tormented pseudosophistication of confused values, it is desirable to recognize that the age of innocence is not necessarily the age of ignorance. Children understand a great deal more than they know. In a world of adult selfishness and injustice, they hug their own secrets to themselves, and retire into a world of fantasy far richer, often enough, than that inhabited by their tormentors. It is the very innocence of the child that constitutes such a fertile soil for the growth of knowledge and understanding. There is nothing that children need be kept in ignorance of. The self-discipline children should be taught—and which they relish—is the best bulwark against having their knowledge run away with them.

An unhurried childhood, rich in varieties of experience, which recognizes the uniqueness of each child, is what the child requires. As humans this is how we are designed to grow and develop.

If I do not dwell here upon the needs of the adolescent and the young and middle-aged adult, it is because their needs are much the same as those of the child, at somewhat more complex levels of integration. At each age the person needs time and space in which to grow and develop. At every age we need the interstimulation of sympathetic others to keep growing in young-spiritedness, and to avoid succumbing to the prevailing mythology of aging.

The tradition of fables we have inherited concerning aging is so old that in many quarters those fables are accepted as truths beyond refutation. Such myths constitute striking examples of the self-fulfilling prophecy. Senility is a disease—it is not an inevitable consequence of aging. Physical, physiological, and psychological changes do occur with aging. There is a great deal of variability in this as between different individuals, depending in part upon genetic and in part upon environmental factors. There is, however, no necessary covariation between the aging of the body and the aging of the mind, any more than there is between chronological aging and aging of different organs. It is unsound, in any event, to infer from the aging body what the state of the mind may be. A feeble, aged body may house a very lively, active mind. The emphasis of the evidence is that we are designed to grow young with the years—not younger, but to retain and develop the qualities of youthfulness that are characteristic of the child. All the available evidence indicates that the best means of retaining that youthfulness is to cultivate the neotenous traits of the child. Aging has been defined as an altered capability for adaptation. There is every reason to believe that with the proper cultivation of those neotenous needs with which we are all endowed, the capabilities for adaptation would be enhanced rather than diminished. Aging is not to be viewed as an accumulation of deficits and losses. What is now well established is that the gains in cognitive functioning, in wisdom, are considerable. It has also been established that up to the age of seventy or thereabouts heredity seems to play a most influential role in the aging of the body; after that it is mainly a matter of habits, individual lifestyle, and personal conduct that favors survival. So, to a significant extent, longevity and the quality of health are conditions that are within our control. That is the main conclusion of all studies devoted to the matter, to wit: that our personal health must be our personal responsibility, and not something we leave to the physician.

The maintenance and increase in intellectual power in the absence of disease is principally dependent upon the continuous exercise of mind. Intellectual activity is as necessary to the healthy development of the mind as is breathing to the healthy development of the lungs.

Recent research indicates that intellectual ability does not decrease through the eighth decade, and that with exercise and training significant gains can be achieved. To remain intellectually active, intellectual stimulation is necessary, and that is what the quality of youthfulness, when it is retained and developed, is constantly encouraging: to remain in touch with reality, to soak up from the environment those nourishing excitations for which the mind hungers and is never quite satiated. All this and more the neotenous mind is designed to secure. All research supports the view that lifetime experiences and exercise of the mind play a basic role in securing and preserving a lively mind into old age. This is especially borne out by the fact that academic men and women, scientists, and thinkers of every kind, seldom exhibit any real falling off in intellectual ability with age.

The later years can be the happiest of one's life. As we have seen, many of those who have achieved what others call "old age" have confessed to feeling embarrassingly young, as if such feeling were something anachronistic, an unexpected freshness. It is the kind of freshness that the long-distance runner experiences when, at the apex of fatigue, he experiences a second wind, which takes him on to the finishing line in a burst of renewed energy. It is the kind of freshness that can be maintained throughout life, and while one is best trained in it in childhood and youth, it is not too late to recapture it in one's later years. The earlier, however, one has been encouraged in one's neotenous qualities, the more likely is one to realize the feeling of unadulterated joy in being alive the romping child so gloriously feels, that gaiety of spirit that has enabled one to grow young more effectively and more happily than was ever before possible—the last of life, for which the first was made.

Appendix A

The historian is a prophet looking backwards.
—SCHLEGEL

A HISTORY OF NEOTENY

New ideas usually have a history. The full understanding of a scientific idea, its ramifications, applications, and significance, generally has to wait on the development of a context into which it can be fitted. So it has been with the idea of neoteny. The term was coined in 1884 by Julius Kollmann, Professor of Zoology at the University of Basel, to describe the process of transformation whereby newts and similar animals mature sexually while still in the larval form. Kollmann cited the axolotl, the aquatic larval stage of the American salamander, as a representative form. This creature was once believed to belong not only to a distinct genus and species, but even more distinctively to a different family (from the salamanders), which went by the grand name of *Siredon axolotl pisciforme.* But in 1867 the French naturalist Auguste Duméril astonished the scientific world by showing that the axolotl was in fact the sexually mature larval form of the salamander then called *Amblystoma,* now known as *Ambystoma.*

Duméril showed that as long as the axolotl continues in its aquatic environment it retains its gills, gill-slits, tail, and aquatic habits, failing altogether to undergo metamorphosis into the terrestrial adult form. When, however, it is transplanted to land or is fed thyroid extract, the axolotl will frequently change into full adult form, and from a gill-breathing aquatic creature is transformed into an entirely lung-breathing terrestrial salamander. There are other newts who will under similar conditions undergo the same kind of metamorphosis. The important point is that the larva will become sexually mature while otherwise remaining permanently in the larval state. It is this phenomenon that Kollmann dubbed neoteny.

Here let me indulge in a little etymological criticism. Kollmann

225

coined the term neoteny by joining the Greek words *neos,* youth, and *teino,* for which, writing in German, he gave the meaning of what he thought to be the German equivalents, *halten, hinhalten,* words that mean "to retain," "delay." Here Kollmann seems to have confused *teino* or *teinein* with the Latin *tenere,* "to hold," for by no stretch of the imagination can *teino* be held to mean anything other than "to stretch, to extend toward." But if Kollmann's etymology was not up to scratch it was nevertheless "well-found," for neoteny is, in fact, both the stretching out and the retention of early traits into sexual maturity or adult life. In other words, one becomes adult while retaining ancestral, larval, fetal, juvenile, or youthful traits, instead of growing old by developing older traits. For our purposes we can best think of neoteny as the time-extension in development of youthful traits— "youthful" here being used in its very broadest sense.

Karl von Baer, Hans Gadow

In 1866 the German embryologist Karl von Baer (1792–1876) had suggested the term *paedogenesis,* from the Greek *paedo,* child, and *genesis,* generation, to designate the condition in which the larval form develops precocious sexual maturity while the remainder of the body is still in the condition of a larva or even an embryo. Von Baer had no notion of the importance for evolution of the retention or stretching out of juvenile traits into adult life. He was merely concerned with the description of the sexually mature larva. The importance of his observation lay in the fact that he recognized, apparently for the first time, that different organ-systems could, in the same organism, develop at very different rates. In modern biology this phenomenon is termed *heterochrony* (Gr. *hetero,* different + *chronos,* time).

More attention was paid to von Baer's observations on heterochronic development than to the term, paedogenesis, he employed to describe it. During the nineteenth and twentieth centuries studies were published on the phenomenon in the world's scientific periodicals mainly on such creatures as insects, toads, frogs (Anura), newts and salamanders (Urodeles). By the beginning of the twentieth century heterochronic development was by most investigators identified as neoteny, and in the standard textbook of the day, Hans Gadow's *Amphibia and Reptiles,* published in 1901, Chapter Three opens with a full discussion of neoteny and concludes that the forms that retain their gills as sexually mature adults are the oldest members of the urodeles. It is in Gadow's book that the term "neoteny" makes its first appearance in an English work. In describing certain metamorphosing amphibia Hadow writes, "These cases are therefore instances of more or less complete retardation, or of the retention of partially larval conditions."

"Retardation," as used by Gadow and others, it should be understood, does not refer to anything abnormal or defective, but simply to perfectly normal heterochronic development.

Edwin Drinker Cope

The great American paleontologist and biologist Edwin Drinker Cope (1840–1897), Professor of Geology at the University of Pennsylvania, without giving it a name recognized the importance of neoteny as a factor of evolution. In an article on "The Origin of Genera," published in 1868, Cope endeavored to show that while natural selection was quite a valid explanation, it was not quite sufficient to account for evolution. Cope maintained that there was an additional mechanism at work. This he called the law of acceleration and retardation. Cope's purpose was to show that "while natural selection operates by the 'preservation of the fittest,' retardation and acceleration act without any reference to 'fitness' at all; that, instead of being controlled by fitness, it is the controller of fitness." Cope went on to suggest that perhaps all the characteristics supposed to mark generalized groups, from genera up, evolved by acceleration and retardation, combined with some intervention by natural selection, and that specific characters or *species* have been evolved by a combination of a lesser degree of acceleration and retardation with a greater degree of natural selection.

Darwin read this article, and in the sixth edition of *The Origin of Species* (1872) drew attention to Cope's law of acceleration and retardation, and observed that "if the age for reproduction were retarded, the character of the species, at least in its adult state, would be modified; nor is it improbable that the previous and earlier stages of development would in some cases be hurried through and finally lost." Darwin goes on to add, "Whether species have often or ever been modified through this comparatively sudden mode of transition, I can form no opinion; but if this has occurred, it is probable that the differences between the young and the mature, and between the mature and old, were primordially acquired by graduated steps." This is succinctly put. Referring to this formulation of his theory, Cope later wrote (in 1887) that "it is quite misunderstood by Darwin, as will be sufficiently evident from the following quotation from the last edition of his *Origin of Species*, 1872, p. 149: 'There is another possible mode of transmission, namely, through the acceleration or retardation of the period of reproduction. This has lately been insisted on by Prof. Cope and others in the United States.' " To this Cope added, "This has only been dwelt on as accounting for a very minor grade of differences seen in race and sex."

Cope was correctly referring to the retardation of morphological traits, not as Darwin misunderstood him to say, retardation of the age of reproduction.

In an 1870 essay by Cope on "The Hypothesis of Evolution: Physical and Metaphysical," he wrote,

> The modifications presented by man have, then, resulted from an acceleration in development in some respects, and retardation perhaps in others . . . the characters of the human genus were probably developed successively; but few of the indications of human superiority appeared until the combination was accomplished. . .
>
> "Acceleration" means a gradual increase in the rate of assumption of successive characters in the same period of time. A fixed rate of assumption of characters, with gradual increase in the length of the period of growth, would produce the same result—*viz.*, a longer development scale and the attainment of an advanced position.

And finally,

> The law of anatomy and paleontology is, that we must seek the point of departure of the type which is to predominate in the future, at lower stages on the line, in less decided forms, or in what, in scientific parlance, are called generalized types. In the same way, though the adults of the tailless apes are in a physical sense more highly developed than their young, yet the latter far more closely resemble the human species in their large facial angles and shortened jaws.
>
> How much significance, then, is added to the law uttered by Christ!— "Except ye become as little children, ye can not enter the kingdom of heaven." Submission of will, loving trust, confiding faith—these belong to the child: how strange they appear to the executing, commanding, reasoning

man! Are they so strange to the woman? We all know the answer. Woman is nearer to the point of departure of that development which outlives time and peoples heaven; and if man would find it, he must retrace his steps, regain something he lost in youth, and join to the powers and energies of his character the submission, love and faith which the new birth alone can give.

From this passage it is evident that Cope had clearly grasped the importance of behavioral neoteny for the development of humankind. Yet his ideas on this subject have gone unnoticed for more than a century. But better late, and well found, than never. Cope was a religious man, a Quaker, a great scientist and a towering thinker, a prolific worker and writer, and altogether a remarkable man.

Havelock Ellis

The idea of neoteny, although, again, not the term itself, was independently applied to the development of humankind by that extraordinary genius, humanist, anthropologist, sexologist, and man of letters Havelock Ellis (1859–1939). Ellis will always be remembered for his pioneering and courageous seven-volume *Studies in the Psychology of Sex,* published between 1897 and 1928, a work that did more than any other, before or since, to change attitudes and ideas toward sex.

Ellis, who was apparently not a reader of the literature on the comparative anatomy of newts and frogs and had seemingly not encountered the idea of "neoteny," nevertheless accurately described it in the book he undertook as a preparation for his *Studies in the Psychology of Sex,* entitled *Man and Woman,* first published in 1894, and in many editions subsequently. It remains a marvelous source book, and a most readable one, on its subject. In this work Ellis clearly recognized the importance of neoteny, without giving it a name, as a factor in the evolution of humans and in the differentiation of the sexes. Comparing ape and human fetuses with their adult forms, Ellis wrote,

The Ape starts in life with a considerable human endowment, but in the course of life falls far away from it; Man starts in life with a still greater portion of human or ultra-human endowment, and to a less extent falls from it in adult life, approaching more and more to the Ape.

We might say that the foetal evolution which takes place sheltered from the world is in an abstractly upward direction. . . . We see, therefore, that the infantile condition in both Apes and Man is somewhat alike and approximates to the human condition.

It seems that up to birth, or shortly afterwards, in the higher mammals such as the Apes and Man, there is a rapid and vigorous movement along the line of upward zoological evolution, but that a time comes when this foetal or infantile development ceases to be upward, but is so directed as to answer to the life wants of the particular species.

"The human infant," Ellis concluded, "presents in an exaggerated form the chief distinctive characters of humanity—the large head and brain, the small face, the hairlessness, the delicate bony system." To which he adds the trenchant words, "By some strange confusion of thought we usually ignore this fact, and assume that the adult form is more highly developed than the infantile form." Finally, concerning the relative evolutionary status of the sexes, Ellis wrote,

When we have realised the position of the child in relation to evolution we can take a clearer view as to the natural position of woman. She bears the special characteristics of humanity in a higher degree than man . . . simply because she is nearer to the child. Her conservatism is thus compensated and justified by the fact that she represents more nearly than man the human type to which man is approximating. . . . The progress of our race has been a progress in youthfulness.

Ellis appears independently to have arrived at the concept of neoteny, especially as it referred to the evolution of humans and the differentiation of the sexes, but while he evidently regarded the phenomenon as important enough to discuss at length, he failed to give it a name. Had he done so he might have succeeded in drawing attention earlier to the idea, if not to the term, as an important factor in human evolution.

During the first decade of the twentieth century fetal traits as a source of adult features in humans were recognized by a number of biologists.

J. E. V. Boas, Otto Jaekel, Alfred Giard, J. H. F. Kohlbrugge, Adam Sedgwick

In 1896 J. E. V. Boas, a Danish zoologist, devoted an essay to neoteny in which he cited many examples of organisms that exhibited typical neotenous traits, in the form of youthful anatomical features characteristic of ancestral forms prominent in their adult descendants. Boas suggested that the late descent of the testes and the double vagina in some animals were probably examples of neotenous traits.

In 1901 the German zoologist Otto Jaekel, in a discussion of the various ways in which evolution occurs, referred to what are essentially neotenic phenomena as *epistasis*.

Also in 1901 the French zoologist Alfred Giard employed the term *progenesis* to describe paedomorphosis produced by accelerated maturation and precocious truncation of development. In 1908 the German biologist J. H. F. Kohlbrugge in his book on the descent of man discussed a number of examples of fetal traits as the source of adult features in humans.

In 1909 Adam Sedgwick, Professor of Zoology and Comparative Anatomy at Cambridge University, pointed out that contrary to the views of those who held that evolution proceeded by the adding on of newly developed traits at the end of a life-history, the evidence seemed to show that evolution proceeded by modification of stages in the life-history. "Inasmuch," he wrote, "as the organism is variable at every stage of its independent existence and is exposed to the action of natural selection there is no reason why it should escape modification at any stage."

In other words, the development of new traits in the evolution of any species is not necessarily a matter of the addition of novel elements to already existing structures, but rather may occur by modification or changes at any stage during development—or, as we would phrase it today, changes produced by modification of relative growth rates rather than by change of material in the embryo.

Some pages later in the same article, in considering the evolution of living forms in the past, Sedgwick remarked "that what we call organic evolution has consisted in a gradual evolution of new environments to which the organism's innate capacity of change has enabled it to adapt itself. We have warrant for this possibility in the case of the Axolotl and in other similar cases of neoteny."

In other words, the axolotl can adapt itself to an existence in the water or on land, depending on the environment acting upon it. It is the environment that challenges the adaptive capacities of organisms, not the other way round. The organism must adapt itself to such challenges through its genes, and this may involve competition in one form or another between organisms. It is, however, the environment that acts as the selective agent. The uniqueness and variety of environments to which humans have been exposed in the course of their five million or more years of development have resulted in an extraordinary variety of adaptive responses. It is necessary for us to understand such facts if we are to appreciate the role that neoteny has played in human evolution.

Walter Garstang

Surveying the role of evolution throughout the whole of the animal kingdom, Ernst Haeckel (1834–1919), Professor of Zoology at the University of Jena, announced in 1874 what he called the "Law of Recapitulation." This "law" stated that "ontogeny repeats phylogeny"—in its individual development every organism repeats its ancestral history—more precisely, in short, that in embryonic development the successively later structural stages of *adult* ancestral forms or traits are repeated. Hence, in development the organism climbs, as it were, its own family tree. That this theory or "principle," as it came to be known and for many years accepted by zoologists, is today discredited is largely due to the critical examination to which it was subjected in 1922 by the English biologist Walter Garstang, Professor of Zoology at the University of Reading. The facts that Garstang set out before the reader made it clear that the very opposite of Haeckel's "Law of Recapitulation" was true. "Ontogeny," Garstang demonstrated, "does not repeat phylogeny: it creates it." In recapitulation the embryonic descendant is alleged to resemble the adult ancestor; in fact Garstang found the reverse to be true, namely, that the adult descendant resembles the embryonic or fetal ancestor. To describe the process by which this occurred Garstang introduced the term *paedomorphosis* (Gr. *paedo,* child, + *morphosis,* body-formation), meaning "formed like a child."

Garstang defined paedomorphosis as a mechanism whereby evolutionary advance is achieved in certain highly progressive species, including humans, by the retention in the adult of structures formerly found only in the fetal stages of the individuals of the species. This is neoteny, the reverse or opposite of recapitulation.

Biologists and others have sometimes written as if they considered evolution to be the product of a single process such as natural selection, mutation, hybridization, isolation, or genetic drift. This is to misread the meaning of the evolutionary process, how it in fact works. As the distinguished geneticist Theodosius Dobzhansky has said, "Perhaps the most important advance in evolutionary thought was the realization that it is the coaction of many agents that brings about evolutionary changes. What kind of change occurs in a population depends on the magnitudes of all the 'forces' impinging upon it as well as on the genetic structure of the population determined by its previous history."

Among the factors coacting to bring about evolutionary change, perhaps the most underestimated has been neoteny or paedomorphosis. From a genetic and developmental point of view—that is, taking into consideration both the genetic facts and developmental processes—one can readily understand how a specialized race of animals may escape from specialization. All that is necessary is that such a group of animals be characterized by a less or differently specialized larval or juvenile form. Genes controlling rates of development will then make possible retardation or acceleration of development, and hence evolutionary change, as well as the avoidance of specialization.

The genetic changes, however, must occur in the early stages of development in the embryo, larva, or fetus. As Sir Arthur Keith (1866–1955), English anthropologist and Conservator of the Royal College of Surgeons, put it in a lecture delivered in 1923, "Man's outstanding structural peculiarities have been produced during the embryonic and foetal stages of his evolutionary history." And again, in 1925, "The intrauterine period gives every opportunity for the working out of new inventions."

Given such an adaptable genetic system and a sufficient amount of time, animal stocks may by such paedomorphic processes escape from the path of extinction. As A. C. Hardy, Professor of Zoology at Oxford University and son-in-law of Walter Garstang (who toppled "The Law of Recapitulation,"), put it,

In the great majority of stocks the end must come before this rare opportunity of paedomorphosis can intervene; but in a very small minority the

chance comes earlier, before it is too late, and such lines are switched by
selection to new pathways with fresh possibilities of adaptive radiation. So
vast is the span of time available, that, rare as they may be, these escapes
from specialization seem likely to have provided some of the more fundamental innovations in the course of evolution.

Louis Bolk

Perhaps the most influential writer on neoteny as a factor in human
evolution was Louis Bolk (1866–1930), Professor of Anatomy at the
University of Amsterdam. Bolk began writing on the subject as early as
1914. In a work published that year on the formation of the teeth in the
monkeys, apes, and humans—the primates—Bolk drew attention to the
small size of the teeth in humans, the occasional loss of the upper
lateral incisors, the third molars, and the frequent persistence of the
mandibular deciduous molar in the lower jaw. These conditions, Bolk
pointed out, approximate more closely to the fetal than to the adult
stages of human development.

Bolk had been thinking for a good many years about the mechanisms
involved in the retention of fetal traits in the adult human, but it was not
until early in 1921, in a lecture (somewhat awkwardly entitled "On the
Character of Morphological Modifications in Consequence of Affec-
tions of the Endocrine Organs") delivered to the Dutch Academy of
Sciences in Amsterdam, that he presented the theory that is today
associated with his name. It is an idea, he tells us, that he had thought
about for years, but that he had never really been able to correlate
adequately with other views or observations. At last he found the solution in the role he believed the endocrine glands, or glands of internal
secretion, played in bringing about specific morphological evolutionary
changes. Citing such features as the relative hairlessness of humans,
the late closure of the cranial sutures, the absence of brow ridges, the
vertical face and nonprojecting jaws (orthognathy), Bolk went on to
show how the development of such traits is controlled by the endocrine
glands in pathological and abnormal conditions.

It was at this time that Bolk put forward what he knew would strike
his listeners as a rather strange idea, namely the concept of retardation.
"I propose to demonstrate," he said, "that the development of the
specifically human characteristics is the result of a retardative or sup-

pressing activity of the endocrine organs." He added, "I hope further to draw your attention to phenomena from which we may conclude that the retardative influence not only concerns the merely morphological faculties, but that the entire process of development, the developmental rate of the human individual, as compared with that of other Primates, is retarded."

In this lecture Bolk also referred to the role the endocrines had probably played in the evolution of the human species. In the same year (1921) he published an article in the leading English medical journal, *The Lancet*. There followed in rapid succession a series of articles from Bolk's pen that indicated the serious thought, experiment, and observation he was devoting to endocrinogenous retardation. In an article published in 1923, "On the Significance of the Supraorbital Ridges in the Primates," he argued that the absence in humans of these brow ridges—which are so pronounced in adult apes—is a fetal feature. "All typical human somatic properties," Bolk wrote, "are persisting fetal features."

In the same year Bolk published an article on "The Problem of Orthognathism," that is, on the somewhat vertical or flattish face of humans compared with other primates; this, he showed, represented a persisting fetal feature. In 1924, in an article on "The Chin Problem," the same claim was made for that unique feature of the human lower jaw, the projecting chin.

In 1925 Bolk employed the term "fetalization" to refer to the process of retention of fetal traits into adulthood. This he did in a lecture entitled "The Problem of Anthropogenesis," delivered before the Dutch Academy of Sciences in December 1925, and published in its *Proceedings* in 1926. Here Bolk makes his primary point: "For where," he writes, "present-day Man may be bodily considered as a Primate-fetus that has become sexually mature, our ancestors already possessed all our specific properties, though only as temporary developments, by way of transitional stage. This is the principle of what I term the *Fetalization-theory* of Anthropogeny."

In April 1926 Bolk delivered the same lecture to the Anatomical Society at Freiburg. Later in the same year, somewhat enlarged, the lecture was published as a forty-four-page pamphlet, *Das Problem der Menschwerdung*. In this work, which has undoubtedly been the most widely influential and most often quoted of all his writings, Bolk presented his "new theory" concerning the evolution of humankind, arguing that "fetalization cannot have resulted from external influences acting upon the organism." Contrary to Darwin, he maintained that human morphology was not the effect of an adaptation to modified external conditions, that "it was not brought about under the influence of a struggle for life, it was not the result of natural or sexual selection, for these evolutional factors exert their influence not on the body as a whole but in a more limited way, on circumscribed parts of the organism." Bolk here clearly seems to have been among the first to understand the fact of mosaic evolution (see Chapter One). Bolk went on to say that he saw anthropogenesis—that is to say the evolution of man—as the effect of a single functional process, the retention in the adult of prehuman fetal or infant traits. These early stages, he argued, were retained by developmental arrests or retardations—in other words, the process of "fetalization."

These are important points, for while Bolk was an anti-Darwinian, his conception of fetalization actually fits perfectly into the Darwinian schema, or at least into the neo-Darwinian biology of today.

Bolk appears to have been one of the earliest biologists to emphasize that not all evolution occurs by adaptation to the environment. Biologists today understand that evolutionary change may occur through accidental changes in fecundity, as a result of which a population with a higher reproductive rate may replace one with a lower reproductive rate. In addition, such changes may occur as a result of differential growth (allometry—Gr. allo, various + metro, measure), the relative growth of part of an organism in comparison with the whole. Different parts of the body grow at different rates, and these rates of growth vary considerably among different members of the order of animals to which humans belong, the primates. The human brain, for example, grows much more rapidly in relation to the body than does the ape brain. Among primates the brain, after birth, grows at a slower rate than the body, small primates tending to have a proportionately larger brain than the great apes. There are a number of other respects in which the differential growth of the parts of the body in different primates cannot be explained on adaptive grounds.

Traits may become established in a species simply as a result of the fact that one of the effects of a gene may be carried along by the organism because of another of its effects, which was the one that was naturally selected for its adaptive value. For example, a gene for an enzyme that has been selected for its detoxifying effects upon poisonous substances may also effect skin color change, which may have no adaptive value whatever. Such various effects of a single gene, is known as *pleiotropy* (Gr. *pleion,* more + *tropos,* turning). Similarly, an unselected gene genetically linked with one undergoing selection may be carried along with the latter and express itself in some non-adaptive trait. This is known as "the hitchhiker effect."

Bolk was ahead of his time in seeing that neoteny, which he called "fetalization," primarily was a matter of developmental rather than adaptive change. A principal defense of the manner in which neotenous changes were produced in humans does not depend upon their adaptive value. Simple developmental causes are quite sufficient to explain such things as the flat-facedness of humans, the presence of a developed chin, the shape of the skull, loss of pigment, and many other neotenous traits. Such traits, however, while not the result of natural selection, may nevertheless indirectly be of adaptive value. The reduction in the size of the eyeteeth (canines), however it came about, led to the elimination of the spaces in the jaws into which the tips of these teeth had formerly been received. The reduction of these spaces (diastemata) resulted in a flattening of the face. The large brain may constitute another example. Size of brain is certainly a neotenous trait, but size in itself is not the important thing. What *are* of importance are the potentialities, the arrangements within the brain that, under certain conditions, render human development possible. But then again, most of those arrangements are almost certainly due to natural selection, even though the size of the brain in which they have their being may not be.

PRIMARY HUMAN CHARACTERISTICS
In support of his fetalization theory Bolk presented the following list of primary human characteristics preserved in adult humans:

Flat-facedness (orthognathy)
Reduction or lack of body hair
Loss of pigment in skin, eyes, and hair
Form of external ear
Epicanthic eyefold (median eyelid skinfold)
Central position of the major opening, the foramen magnum, at base of skull
High brain weight
Persistence of cranial sutures to advanced age

Structure of hands and feet
Persistence of labia majora
Downward orientation of vagina
Form of pelvis
Specific variations of the dentition and cranial sutures

When these primary characteristics of humans are considered in the light of individual primate development, it is found, said Bolk, that they show one common characteristic, namely that in humans the common primate fetal condition has become permanent. In other words, traits that in individual development in other primates are transitory, in humans are retained. Development in humans, Bolk declared, is conservative; in apes it is propulsive. Insofar as form is concerned, what in apes represents a passage from one developmental stage to another has become a terminal stage in humans.

At this point in his discussion Bolk comments on an issue he was to develop later, that the terms he applies to the development of nonhuman primates and to humans may also be applied to the differences existing between races.

The answer, then, says Bolk, to the question What is the essential difference between human and ape? is simply: the fetal character of human form. This leads us to a view, says Bolk, that renders it unnecessary to deduce the specific characteristics of the human body from those of other primates. Humans in their bodies have preserved their ancestral fetal traits, whereas the apes have gone on to develop the *adult* bodily traits of their ancestors. "If," wrote Bolk, "I wished to express the basic principle of my ideas in a somewhat strongly worded sentence, I would say that man, in his bodily development, is a primate fetus that has become sexually mature."

To the known factors of evolution, Bolk claimed, a new one must be added: retardation of development. No mammal grows at so slow a rate as the human. The essential characteristic of the human as organism is the slow tempo of development. This Bolk distinguished as the principle of retardation, of becoming human—anthropogenesis. Thus, human form is the result of retardation. The process of retardation, Bolk felt, was principally the consequence of hormonal influences. This he thought one could perceive in comparing the remains of extinct hominids back to the earliest ancestral forms. Paleolithic humans developed faster—that is, achieved full growth at an earlier age—than modern humans. Thus the eruption of the teeth in Neandertals, he found, followed an anthropoid pattern; their teeth also erupted earlier. Furthermore, Bolk pointed out, the male matures sexually at a slower rate than the female. All this Bolk saw as the work of the endocrine glands, whose secretions in the form of hormones acted to produce differentiation of the bodily structures. It so happened that during the period in which Bolk was writing the hormones and their effects were just beginning to be discovered, so that Bolk was provided with a ready explanation for the means whereby fetalization could be achieved.

While it is true that hormones do play a fundamental role in the slowing-down or acceleration of development, today we know that hormones represent but one of several intermediate steps in the processes involved in the regulation of development. The controlling factors in growth and development are principally genetic—allowing, of course, for the fact that the expression of any trait is almost always the result of the interaction between genes or genetic developmental schedules and the environments with which they interact. It is the fact, however, that genes regulate the temporal and quantitative expression of the hormones. This was not clear at the time when Bolk wrote. Bolk was quite wrong in bracketing the pattern of eruption of the teeth in Neandertals with the rate at which they erupted in the apes. The teeth in the Neandertals erupted in the same order and at about the same ages as in modern humans. Also, while he was correct in stating that the male develops sexually at a slower rate than the female, he was wrong—and this is where his male chauvinism was undoubtedly showing—in asserting that sexual development is more prolonged in the male than in the female. Reproductive ability is more prolonged in males, but the capacity for sex and orgasm continues in the female into old age much more often than in the male. Menarche (the first menstruation) may occur earlier in the female than spermatogenesis in the male, but first ovulation (which does not coincide with menarche) occurs later in the female than spermatogenesis in the male.

When Bolk goes on to tell us that it is generally known that the rates of development apparently differ among the various "races," and that the "yellow-skinned races" are the most intensely retarded, that is, the most fetalized, he makes an important observation that raises many equally important questions, which even at this date have been far from adequately explored.

M. R. Drennan

In his booklet *A Short Course on Physical Anthropology,* published in
1927, M. R. Drennan, Professor of Anatomy at the University of Cape
Town, ably managed within its sixty pages tò refer to the "arrest of
development with the retention of more youthful phases" as undoubtedly playing "a part in the evolution of new human races—particularly
the dwarf races of mankind." In this little book and in a later article
Drennan employed the concept of neoteny to explain the strikingly
large brains of the extinct African humans known as Boskop man, as
well as many of the features of their presumed descendants, the
Bushmen or Khoi San of South Africa.

O. H. Schindewolf

In 1929 German paleontologist O. H. Schindewolf published an article
of some fifty pages in which he presented an elaborate and convincing
discussion of the role played by neoteny in the evolution of humankind,
a theme which he developed further in his book on paleontology, which
appeared in 1936.

Gavin de Beer

If there is one man who was responsible for making the concept of
neoteny or paedomorphism scientifically respectable it is Gavin de
Beer (1892–1972), Professor of Embryology, University College, University of London, and later Director of the British Museum (Natural
History). In 1930 he published a book entitled *Embryology and Evolution.* In this important and delightful work he discussed the process of
neoteny as observed in animals from insects to humans. In 1940 the
book underwent a change of title to *Embryos and Ancestors,* and under
that title it was subsequently published in two revised editions in 1951
and 1958. De Beer brilliantly showed that the evidence of natural history strongly led to the conclusion that the paedomorphic mode of
evolution is correlated with the appearance of large, successful, and
progressive groups of the animal kingdom. In the evolution of humans,
he pointed out, there seemed to be a progressive increase in the number

of physical traits affected by neoteny, and he argued that the potential for further evolution will remain as long as we retain our neotenous traits—a conclusion of momentous import.

J. B. S. Haldane

Among the outstanding minds of the twentieth century, John Broadus Sanderson Haldane (1892–1964) was surely one of the most extraordinary. He was so many-faceted in his knowledge that he might almost be said to have been globular: classical scholar, mathematician, biochemist, biologist, geneticist, anthropologist, political activist, essayist, eccentric, and much else—there is nothing that he touched in the realm of science that he did not illuminate. His contributions to mathematical genetics and the mathematical foundations of evolutionary theory have had a most powerful influence upon modern evolutionary biology. It is not surprising, then, that Haldane, with his far-ranging mind, should have perceived the importance of neoteny as a factor in the evolution of humankind.

Haldane had read both Bolk and de Beer and been much influenced by them. In his book *The Causes of Evolution,* published in 1932, Haldane points out that the fact that we belong to an order of mammals most of whose members produce a single offspring at birth (monotocous) made possible the establishment of mutations favoring fetalization. In animals that produce several young at a birth (polytocous), intrauterine competition for nourishment and space is considerable. Under such conditions adaptive advantage lies with rapid development, and the emergence of fetalization becomes impossible because genes favoring a slowing-down of development would be eliminated. With one offspring per birth the case is quite different, and a retardation of development becomes a great advantage. The longer the single offspring is preserved in the womb, the more leisurely its development can be, and the more likely it is to be preserved for the species. A fetus in the womb is, on the whole, better nourished and less exposed to danger than a newborn infant.* Under the conditions of life of our precursors and of early

---

* The mode of reproduction characterized by large litters—rapid development, short gestation, and the birth of relatively undeveloped young—is known as *altricial.* The mode of reproduction characterized by small litters—slow development, extended gestation, and the birth of relatively well developed capable young—is known as *precocial.*

forms of humankind, such a prolongation of the intrauterine period of development would have been of great advantage to the fetus. Genes, therefore, favoring such a prolongation of intrauterine development by a slowing down of the rate of fetal development would gradually, by natural selection, have been established as part of the human genetic constitution.

Haldane's observations are most apt. It is reasonably clear that an extended protected period in the environment of the womb would contribute both to a slowing-down of the prenatal rate of development and to a continued postnatal retardation in developmental rate. The slow-down in the prenatal rate should prevent the conceptus from growing too big. It is no argument against this suggestion that the gestation period of the great apes and of humans is of about the same duration, varying from genus to genus by a few weeks more or less. Haldane does not suggest that it is the long period spent in the womb that is the cause of retardation of developmental rates in humans, but that it is a factor that would favor continued variation in that direction. That variation has, indeed, occurred in humans, but not in apes. The apes start out well enough, but rapidly develop gerontomorphic traits, unlike the paedomorphic development of the human. And this applies to their behavioral as well as morphological traits.

The fact that ape and human embryos are more alike than adults merely means that the genes that determine the differences between ourselves and the apes come into action rather later in our life cycle.

Haldane saw slow development as the major evolutionary trend in humans. He underscored the fact that the essential feature of the last stage of human evolution has been not the acquisition of new features but rather the preservation of embryonic and infantile traits that had been developed at a period in the life cycle when the individual was in the womb and sheltered from any form of violence. The retention of these features, Haldane suggested, enabled humans to shed much of their animalism.

"If human evolution continued in the same direction as in the immediate past," Haldane concluded, "the superman of the future would develop more slowly than we, and be teachable for longer. He would retain in maturity some characteristics which most of us lose in childhood. Certain shades of the prison house would never close about him. He would probably be more intelligent than we, but distinctly less staid and solemn."

Olaf Stapledon

In a novel, *First and Last Men,* which in 1930, when it was published, achieved a considerable readership, the author, Olaf Stapledon, told the story of humankind millions of years hence. The "last men" of his novel have evolved in remarkable ways both physically and mentally. To come to maturity takes two thousand years. In addition to being very likable creatures they are characterized by the perfection of their intellectual and moral qualities, and enjoy life, in every way, to the fullest.

Julian Huxley

Julian Huxley, Honorary Lecturer in Zoology at the University of London, in his book *Problems of Relative Growth,* published in 1932, emphasized that the rate of genes controlling development may vary in either a plus or minus direction, accelerating or retarding the processes they affect. In the former case a condition that used to occur in the adult is now run through at an earlier stage. In the latter case a condition that once characterized an earlier phase of development is now shifted to the adult phase. Neoteny, Huxley emphasized, is the most striking example of this effect. Single traits also behave in this way, not simply generalized developmental changes. When this occurs, Huxley illuminatingly remarks, previous adult traits, though still in a real sense potentially present, never appear, because their formation is too long delayed: They are lost to the species by being driven off the time-scale of its development. This is an important point to which we shall return shortly.

Aldous Huxley

Aldous Huxley, novelist and younger brother of Julian, made the idea of neoteny a central theme of his novel *After Many a Summer Dies the Swan,* published in 1939. The title is derived from Tennyson's poem *Tithonus:*

> The woods decay, the woods decay and fall,
> The vapours weep their burthen to the ground,

> Man comes and tills the field and lies beneath,
> And after many a summer dies the swan.

It appears that Julian had mentioned to Aldous that carp in Scottish waters that had been tagged a century earlier were still flourishing. He had also read and heard Julian speak on neoteny, and this, combined with his experience of the Californian preoccupation with death and rejuvenescence, provided him with a ready-made scenario that he had only to fill out in his own uniquely clever way. It appears that in the eighteenth century the Fifth Earl of Gonister had made the discovery that the eating of carp's intestines delayed death. When, in the 1930s, owing to the accidental discovery of a diary the earl had kept, he was discovered in a remote chamber of his castle, he was two hundred years old. But he had lived too long, and the joke was on him. His body was now covered with a mass of coarse red hair; above the matted hair that concealed his jaws and face the eyes stared out of cavernous sockets. There were no eyebrows, just a great ridge of bone, which projected like a shelf under the dirty wrinkled skin. The Fifth Earl of Gonister had grown into an adult fetal ape!

Huxley's preposterous novel is intended to be just that. The ending is, of course, nonsense, but it makes, and was intended to make, a moral point: namely, that when humanity tries to accelerate or retard the pace of development it is in danger of debasing itself. In the sick society, the unregenerate world of cheapened spirituality and *ersatz* values that he saw everywhere about him in Los Angeles, where he had gone to live in 1937, the only hope he could see for humanity lay within the power of each to change himself, and thus change the world.

Frederic Wood Jones, L. Cuénot, and Franck Bourdier

Frederic Wood Jones, perhaps the most brilliant and original anatomist of the twentieth century, in 1938 wrote an essay entitled "Man, Nature's Baby," which was published in the English medical journal *The Lancet,* and later in a book. As a first-rate comparative anatomist particularly interested in the evolution of humans, surveying the evidence, Wood Jones could come to no other conclusion than that the physical makeup of *Homo sapiens* is "that of a singularly immature and undeveloped mammal."

L. Cuénot, distinguished French zoologist, in a 1945 article on neotenic man gave a comprehensive account of the evolution of human physical traits by neoteny. In an article published in 1948 a French prehistorian, Franck Bourdier, considers admixture between "races," fossil man, "juvénisme," and the climatic changes during which much of human evolution occured, all in relation to neoteny and the differentiation of the varieties of humankind.

Gavin de Beer Continues His Missionary Work on Behalf of Neoteny

Probably the best account of the role played by neoteny or paedomorphism in the evolution of humankind was written by Gavin de Beer and published in 1948 in the Festschrift volume honoring distinguished paleontologist Robert Broom. This was entitled "Embryology and the Evolution of Man." In this essay de Beer developed the theme that paedomorphosis allows for the possibility of evolution of traits "clandestinely," in the young stages of a phylogenetic line, the changes becoming revealed when the adult stages are discarded. The sudden appearance of new types, and the apparent gaps in phylogenetic series, receive a logical explanation on these lines. This, incidentally, provides an explanation for the absence of transitional forms.

Since the paedomorphic mode of evolution enables ancestral specializations to become discarded and lost, de Beer makes it clear that by this means new trends of evolution can be superimposed upon the old, and that if this is so then there can be no justification for regarding the mere possession of brow ridges in Neandertal man as disqualifying that stock from having given rise to modern humans. As de Beer points out, the fossil evidence fully supports the view that the evolution of modern humans occurred by paedomorphosis from a Neandertaloid stock and the retention of youthful traits with consequent discarding of Neandertaloid features. The evidence presented by such young Neandertal skulls as were then known all lacked heavy brow ridges, presenting a condition from which modern humans could without difficulty have been derived.

By way of illustration of the importance of paedomorphosis in incorporating modern humans traits that were embryonic or youthful in our ancestors, de Beer cites Devaux's interesting observation that the movable rosey everted lips of humans can best be understood as an adaptation to prolonged suckling and must have originated at an infantile stage. Their retention in adult life, beyond the period of their original usefulness, is to serve as accessory feeding organs, and de Beer suggests that their present function of kissing may have been of considerable importance in sexual selection.

In a BBC broadcast delivered in December 1950 entitled "Peter Pan Evolution," de Beer called the delaying processes of neoteny "The Peter Pan" effect. He pointed out that in the course of evolution, those groups in which evolutionary novelties originated in the adult stages, that is, by gerontomorphism, are precisely the groups that have made the least progress. By contrast, those in which evolutionary novelties originated in the young stages, are precisely the groups in which evolutionary progress has been most marked. De Beer remarks, "Perhaps there is no reason to be surprised at this, for it is a well-established maxim that if great effects are to be produced, it is necessary to start early." Evolution by neoteny or paedomorphosis, de Beer added, may be likened to a rejuvenating effect. And that, indeed, is what its effect is. Evolving by neoteny and having moved into a new zone of adaptation, namely the human-made environment or culture, it has become essential to maintain and progressively reinforce this paedomorphic effect.

In London in 1959, at the Fifteenth International Congress of Zoology, over which de Beer had the honor of presiding, he contributed an illuminating address on paedomorphosis. In this, among other things, he drew attention to the fact that the selective value of paedomorphosis in humans has lain in the delay of development, which made a more complex and larger brain possible, while the prolongation of childhood, accompanied by extended parental care and instruction consequent upon memory-stored and speech-communicated experience, allowed humans to benefit from a more efficient apprenticeship for the conditions of life. In his book *Embryos and Ancestors* (1958), de Beer observed, but did not further develop the view, that "Not only physical characters but types of behaviour and mental traits may be susceptible of paedomorphosis and generontomorphosis." Writing as an embryologist and morphologist de Beer did not consider it within his province to carry the discussion beyond the borders of structural development, although in the passage quoted from his Congress address he appears to have been conscious of the fact that neoteny may have played a role in the development of human behavior. It is to be regretted that de Beer did not express himself more fully on the subject.

Finally, in his superb *Atlas of Evolution,* published in 1964, de Beer discusses and illustrates the workings of paedomorphosis as a factor in evolution. Here he explains that during development from the fertilized egg to the adult, the organism is changing continuously, and during that time the genes controlling development react with the environment to synthesize the chemical substances that result in the differentiation of the various organs and tissues. This means that individuals can vary at any time and at any stage in the amount of change or development that they have undergone. It is this potentiality for variability that constitutes the physical basis for neoteny or paedomorphosis. But, as de Beer states, in all matters of natural selection it is the environment that is of paramount importance; as Sir James Gray put it, the organism at every stage of development throws the dice of variation, but the environment calls the winning numbers.

In a striking drawing of the skulls of juvenile and adult apes and fossil and modern humans, de Beer shows how modern adult man with domed skull and vertical forehead without brow ridges can be derived from the series of juvenile fossil forms, but not from that of the adult series (Figure 14). The prolongation of childhood, de Beer observes, also had results of great importance in conferring increased survival benefits on those whose behavior was directed toward the elaboration and consolidation of the bonds between the members of the family, and in conferring survival benefits also upon those children who were capable of accepting authority during the long and vulnerable period of childhood when they were incapable of looking after themselves and lacked experience.

Arnold Gehlen

Arnold Gehlen (1904–1974), German social psychologist, sociologist, and philosophical anthropologist, whose important writings are only just beginning to be translated into English and who until recently has remained unknown among English-speaking behavioral scientists, was fully aware of the importance of neoteny for the development of the human species. In his book *Der Mensch, seine Natur und seine Stellung in der Welt (Man, His Nature and His Place in the World),* which was first

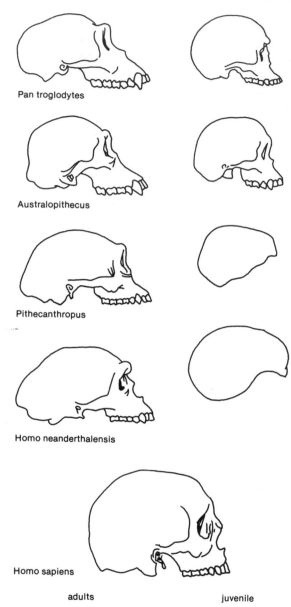

Pan troglodytes

Australopithecus

Pithecanthropus

Homo neanderthalensis

Homo sapiens

adults   juvenile

Fig. 14. Paedomorphosis in the evolution of humans. The right column shows juvenile phases of development, that on the left adult phases of chimpanzee, australopithecine, pithecanthropine, Neandertal, modern adult humans with domed skull, vertical forehead without brow ridges, which can be derived from the series of juvenile forms, but not from that of adult forms. (After de Beer, 1964)

published in 1940 and in nine editions up to 1975, and several times reprinted since then, Gehlen ably discusses the ideas of Bolk and other writers on neoteny. While clearly deeply influenced by these ideas in considering the biological evolution of humankind, Gehlen, however, failed to elaborate on the behavioral consequences of neoteny for humankind. Nevertheless the influence of the idea of neoteny is detectable throughout Gehlen's remarkable book, which is very much worth the reader's attention for its splendid exposition of the nature of human nature.

Konrad Lorenz

In a brilliant study entitled "Part and Parcel in Animal and Human Societies," published in 1950 (in 1971 in English), Konrad Lorenz, the distinguished founder of ethology (the study of animal behavior) and Nobel prize-winner, concluded that "The number of persistent juvenile characters in human beings is so large, and they are so decisive for his overall *habitus,* that I can see no cogent reason for regarding the general juvenescence of man as anything other than a special case of true *neoteny.*" Humans are the creatures whose specialty is nonspecialization, who have remained polymorphously adaptable, free and open to change of every kind. Much influenced by the ideas of Arnold Gehlen's book *Der Mensch* (1940), Lorenz goes on to say, "For anybody who has grasped the fundamental unity and conceptual incomparability of form and function, it will be immediately obvious that the persistence of juvenile behavioural characteristics in man is intimately correlated with that of morphological characters. *The constitutive character of man the maintenance of active, creative interaction with the environment— is a neotenous phenomenon.*" Gehlen's recognition of *the unique human trait of always remaining in a state of development,* Lorenz remarks, "is quite certainly a gift which we owe to the neotenous nature of mankind." This unending state of development is correlated with what Gehlen recognized as man's most important trait, namely the lack of adaptation to a specific environment, which permits humans to be "open to the world" and actively to construct their own environment and surroundings.

Finally Lorenz underscores the point that by far the more important features we should be considering in the investigation of human evolution are not so much physical as behavioral. And here he has much to say that bears upon the future development of humankind, although he mentions a few only of the neotenous behavioral traits of humans.

Weston La Barre

While some have failed to see causal connections and selective forces involved in neoteny, Weston La Barre, Professor of Anthropology at Duke University, in his seminal work *The Human Animal* (1954, suggested that human self-domestication (protection from natural wild enemies, human provision of food, human selective breeding) in the ensuing "trimorphism" of specialization in the male, female, and infant the *enabling factor* is neoteny, that is, the physical specialization of the male (40 percent muscle compared with 23 percent in the female, larger bones and lung capacity, more red blood cells per cubic centimeter) for massive expenditure of energy such as in hunting and protection of the family, within which the (non-hunting) female can specialize in larger-brained, still-not-completed-at-birth single offspring, to which she gives increased and prolonged mammalian care—which in turn allows a dependent neotenous infant time to learn (language, culture, personality). Thus the physical dimorphism of the sexes (ample protection and food-getting, increased female nurturance and care) is in part a response to the single birth (fewer offspring, better care), greatly prolonged intervals between births under dangerously high mortality conditions of rates. But this species-specific sexual dimorphism, developed during the *physical* evolution of humankind, has added to it a species-specific neoteny of the young, which allows the peculiar psychological "humanization" of the species. Since prolonged infancy and childhood puts a burden upon adult animals, neoteny must have been adaptive for the species, with many cultural pasts to borrow from, in place of monolithic instinct.

La Barre regards the nuclear family as a biological and not merely a cultural characteristic of *Homo sapiens*—with prolonged infancy and psychological malleability not only the source of replacement of rigid instinct by cultural *adaptations,* but also the source, first in human beings, of marked human *personality.*

In a later psychoanalytic treatise on religion, La Barre argued that religious cults represent the lingering in a psychic child-status when people dependently anthropomorphize their environment in an inveterately familial model.

In this classical work on the origins of religion, *The Ghost Dance* (1970), La Barre brilliantly examines the enabling factors behind the increasing infantilization of the infant, and concludes that hunting ecology is ultimately behind not only human anatomy but also the human neoteny that is the basis of culture. "For the purposes of the present study," La Barre writes early in his book, "it may be well to emphasize in anticipation the thesis that human neoteny not only provides conditions for learning both of group culture and individual character, *but also forms the experiential matrix for magic and religion, and indeed for the scientific world-view as well.*" The development of this thesis is most fascinatingly carried out by La Barre, opening up a totally new approach to the study of the origins of religion.

It is of interest that La Barre has been the only cultural anthropologist to perceive the importance of neoteny in the evolution of humankind, and to make as much of it as he has done. La Barre clearly saw that neoteny must in some way benefit the *group*, namely through the pooled experience of the group, which transcends knowledge independently obtainable by the individual; hence the adaptive function of a prolonged childhood and youth is to give the creature time enough to learn. "Individual neoteny is the group's way of accumulating and preserving its adaptive lore of past experience."

A. A. Abbie

In 1952 A. A. Abbie, Professor of Anatomy at the University of Adelaide, published a paper entitled "A New Approach to the Problem of Evolution," in which he strongly emphasized the idea that "it is apparent that foetalization underlies most of the major elements characteristic of human evolution. Mere prolongation of the growing period permits an increase in overall dimensions which, up to an optimum which is still uncertain, confers a definite advantage in the struggle for existence." Abbie then asked the question: If all primate fetuses are so much alike, how far back in fetal development must one go to find an indifferent common generalized form that might become any kind of primate? At what stage do such primate fetuses become indistinguishable from one another?

As a working hypothesis Abbie selected an embryo of seven weeks' gestation, as shown in Figure 7 (page 19). As Abbie states, at that stage total development is that of a generalized primate; the digits of the hand are differentiated but those of the feet are not; the great toe could become free and rotated as in apes or fixed (adducted) in series with the other toes as in humans. The ultimate development of the embryo is, of course, already largely determined at conception, but, as Abbie says, it would take only a minor shift in emphasis to produce any variety of primate foot. And without apparently being aware of Keith's earlier statement of the essentially same idea (see Arthur Keith, "The Adaptational Machinery Concerned in the Evolution of Man's Body," *Nature*, 18 August 1923. Supplement.), Abbie stresses that a common ancestry for any or all of the primates is to be sought among primate embryos, not adults.

The point—made many times before—is an important one, namely that neoteny, involving as it does the persistence of early stages of development into later life, enables us to understand and to explain the many otherwise inexplicable gaps that seem to exist between the adult stages of different species, subspecies, varieties, or forms that are clearly closely related.

George Gaylord Simpson

In his book *The Major Features of Evolution* (1953), the American paleontologist George Gaylord Simpson pointed out that some mutant genes affect rates of development and time of termination of development, and that such changes in rate may have distinct or even radical effects on adult form. He echoes de Beer (1930) and Haldane (1932) when he writes that adaptations introduced into juvenile stages that do not affect individual development (caenogenesis) "followed by paedogenesis or neoteny (retardation of development, cessation of development at an earlier stage than in the ancestry, or both) would result in paedomorphosis, appearance of the formerly juvenile characters in the adult. This might seem to be abrupt if the earlier juveniles were unknown and if the neoteny resulted from a single mutation." The reasons, then, why some mutations have small while others have large effects are to be found in the process whereby mutations acquire phenotypic, that is, manifest, expression in the development of the individual.

Ashley Montagu

In 1955 in a paper entitled "Time, Morphology, and Neoteny in the Evolution of Man," I endeavored to explain the appearance of certain modernlike morphological traits in a variety of fossil hominids by the process of neoteny. I also suggested that neotenous changes may have occurred with different, probably insubstantial, frequencies in different early hominid populations derived from a common stock; by this means, in isolated hominid populations, very appreciable morphologic changes could have been brought about.

In 1956 in a paper entitled "Neoteny and the Evolution of the Human Mind," I proposed the theory that the shift from the status of ape to human being was the result of neotenous mutations that produced a retention of the growth trends of the juvenile brain and its potentialities for learning into the adolescent and adult phases of development. It is clear that the nature of those potentialities must also have undergone intrinsic change, for no amount of extension of the chimpanzee's capacity for learning would yield a human mind.

It was further suggested that from the earliest days of human origin evolution by neoteny of the mental capacities had been a gradual process. The progressive increase in the size of the brain, for example, seems to have been paralleled by a progressive increase in mental capacities. Size of brain appears to have stabilized itself in humans; if anything there seems to have been a slight decline in gross size of brain since the days of Neandertal man. This does not, however, mean that the increase in cortical availability has come to an end. Increase in brain cell accommodation has been achieved by the deepening and multiplication of the cerebral convolutions; that is, by increasing the surface area of the brain without increasing its size. I have elsewhere argued that there was no reason to suppose that either the quality or duration of the human capacity for learning will not be subject to further evolution. In various articles published in 1956, 1957, and 1962, and in my books *Introduction to Physical Anthropology* (1960) and *The Human Revolution* (1965) these ideas were further developed.

Theodosius Dobzhansky

Theodosius Dobzhansky (1900–1975), distinguished American geneticist, argued in his classic book *Mankind Evolving* (1962) that fetalization falls short of giving a causal explanation of human evolution. That
is a just judgment and, as Dobzhansky said, it is no disparagement of
the fetalization theory to say that it fails to do so. But, whatever Bolk
may have maintained as to causes, the fact is that the modern theory of
neoteny makes no claim to provide a causal explanation of human
evolution—what it claims is that neoteny is one of the processes or
mechanisms (to use a poor word) by means of which many of the traits
characteristic of humans have been brought into being. It is further
suggested that the means by which the retardative processes have been
effected has been through genes regulating developmental processes, as
shown initially by the work of Ford and Huxley (1927), and subsequently by many other workers. As Huxley has said,

There can be no question that both the relative and absolute rate of developmental processes may be altered genetically, and that such alterations may
have important (as well as trivial) effects on the appearance or disappearance
of characters, and on the pattern of the life-history as a whole. There can
also, I think, be no question that paedomorphosis has played a significant
role in our own evolution. Though it will not account for all the special
characters we possess, notably the special enlargement of the association
areas of our cortex, and the full adaptation of our feet and legs to bipedal
terrestrial existence, it has certainly helped us to escape from anthropoid
specialization.

It is the possibility of escaping from the blind alleys of specialization into a
new period of plasticity and adaptive radiation which makes the idea of
paedomorphosis so attractive in evolutionary theory. Both its possibilities
and limitations deserve the most careful exploration.

Huxley in this passage was commenting on an article by A. C.
Hardy, "Escape from Specialization" (see p. 276), to which we have
already referred. In this article Hardy discussed the views of his father-
in-law, Walter Garstang, on neoteny, arguing that it "is in fact . . . of
cardinal importance in the general process of evolution."

Robert Kuttner

Robert Kuttner, American psychologist, in an article entitled "An Hypothesis on the Evolution of Intelligence," published in 1960, offered the hypothesis that intelligence grew out of instinct, and that fetalization or neoteny was the means by which this development was brought about. Fetalization of brain growth, Kuttner suggested, is correlated with fetalization of brain function. Rigidified instinctive behavior is never developed in humans, as it is in other animals. Since humans are derived from "lower" animals, intelligence must, then, be regarded as an evolutionary derivative of instinct.

Kuttner went on to suggest that intelligence evolved in "higher" species as a consequence of the retention of the behavioral plasticity characteristic of organisms during their immature or larval stages. Very likely. But whatever the case may have been in other animals, instinct as a precursor out of which intelligence developed in humans or in their forerunners is a wholly unnecessary idea. The principle of parsimony or economy in explanation (Ockham's Razor) applies here. It is more likely that natural selection favoring individuals who were adaptively flexible is sufficient to account for the neotenic effect. What can be done with fewer assumptions is done in vain with more.

R. F. Ewer

It is possible to claim too much for neoteny, and in an excellent discussion of this entitled "Natural Selection and Neoteny" (1960), Dr. R. F. Ewer, Lecturer in Zoology at the University of Ghana, has attempted to correct several of the excesses committed by some who have written on the subject. She rightly points out that the failure to consider the selective forces involved in changes that have been attributed to neoteny has led to error. Ewer does not deny the reality of neoteny, or that neotenous processes are "a necessary element in the 'ascent of man,' " but, she claims, they represent merely secondary consequences of the non-paedomorphic key traits. For example, the later members of a phylogenetic series may be expected to have larger brains than earlier ones. In humans the relatively large size of the brain, she says, does not result from a general curtailing of growth.

But this is to misunderstand what is claimed for neoteny. It is not a "curtailing" of growth "so that juvenile proportions are preserved in the adult" (Ewer) that is claimed, but a retention of *the fetal growth rate* during the first years of life, and this is a fact, *not* a theory! Especially during the first postnatal year growth rates maintain the fetal tempo, as Kovács (1960) and others have shown. Insofar as brain size is concerned, the rate of growth characteristic of the fetus is maintained well into the third year (see Table V). The human brain does not represent a return to a juvenile condition, as Ewer thinks the theory of neoteny claims, but represents the culmination of a growth gradient or direction of development, which in its early promise is seen in the juvenile ape brain, arrested in the growing ape, but continued in the growing human.

Ewer's second point is one that cannot be too strongly emphasized; it is that, as Le Gros Clark wrote (1971), "Neoteny is not the cause but rather the concomitant of evolutionary change, for the latter is primarily affected by the selective action of the environment on actively living and breeding populations, as a whole."

Ewer thinks that too much has been made of the relatively small size of the human dentition as an evidence of neoteny, although she admits that the small size of the jaws can be so interpreted. But most investigators agree that both in form and size the dentition of modern man resembles that of the milk teeth of the fossil African apemen, the australopithecines.

The one last point Ewer discusses is "the prolonged period of childhood of man"; she finds it difficult to decide whether this is to be regarded as paedomorphic or not, "since man has not only a longer childhood but also a longer total life-span than other primates." But that is just the point. The total life-span of humans reflects the longer duration of each of their phases of development—infancy, early childhood, later childhood, adolescence, nubility, maturity, and later years—and these are all neotenous, if we are to understand by neoteny the extension of juvenile rates of development into all age phases of subsequent development. "Man," Ewer concludes, "may have escaped from primate arboreal specialization and in so doing found the whole world literally at his feet, but this was done not merely by 'becoming as little children' which, while it may qualify for entry into the Kingdom of Heaven, would have resulted in earthly extinction, had it not been preceded by the acquisition of new characters not present in either the adult or the baby of any other primate."

This is well put, but no one is suggesting that "we become as little children." That, again, is to misunderstand the meaning of neoteny. What neoteny tells us is not that we remain arrested at the level of the fetus or the child, but that we continue to develop the generalized traits that are seen in fetuses and children, rather than become restricted by adult specializations that constrain other primates. As Ewer states, humans have acquired new traits not present in either the adult or juvenile of any other primate. The facts suggest that without natural selection there could be no neoteny, and that not every evolutionary change that has occurred in the evolution of humans is neotenous. Ewer includes complex symbol usage, speech, the erect posture, and everted membranous lips, as examples of new traits, forgetting that everted membranous lips, at any rate, represent a fetal trait. The fact remains that the evolution of some traits by agencies other than neoteny does not make neoteny less a reality of the total evolutionary process. By all means let us avoid the facile and unanalytical application of the label "neoteny" to any and every evolutionary change. In spite of the fact that Bolk almost did, I do not believe that anyone else ever intended such an indiscriminate labeling. However, one must be constantly on one's guard against the kind of enthusiasm for a theory that renders one insensible to the facts.

Mosaic Evolution

What is necessary to understand is that traits in evolution do not develop as harmonious wholes, in a sort of immutable togetherness. As Ernst Mayr has pointed out, every evolutionary type is a mosaic of primitive and advanced characters, of generalized and primitive features. There is an unequal evolution of the components, of the traits, of the type. We are no exception to that rule. Indeed, the evolution of humankind provides a perfect example of mosaic evolution. The development of the erect posture, rearrangement of the pelvic girdle, bipedalism, and freeing of the upper extremities and hands for all the complex functions they were called upon to perform—all this came about well before the increase in the size and complexity of the brain and the remodeling of the skull. As Mayr has stated, mosaic evolution is characteristic of all forms that move into a new adaptive zone; in such conditions one structure or complex of structures is usually under strong selection pressure. "This structure or complex then evolves very rapidly while all others lag behind. As a result there is not a steady and harmonious change of all parts of the 'type,' . . . but rather a 'mosaic evolution.' '' Humankind, it should be added, has continually been moving into new adaptive zones, both physical and humanmade.

Just as in individual development different organs develop at different rates (heterochrony), so in the evolution of a species different organs, different structures, and other traits are characterized by different rates and different degrees of development. Mosaic evolution operates within a variety of different evolutionary matrices to bring forward, by neoteny, the adaptive traits of ancestral juveniles, even when this involves phyletic extension of individual development beyond its ancestral termination, i.e., by hypermorphosis. Examples are increase in body size, increase in length of lower extremities, and increase in complexity of differentiating organs, each an advantageous trait produced in a matrix of retardation.

William A. Mason

William Mason, Professor of Psychology at the University of California at Davis, is an authority on the behavior of apes. In a 1968 article on the effects of early social deprivation on nonhuman primates and their implications for human behavior, Mason asked: Since physical traits are subject to neoteny, might not this also be true of behavior? He suggested that from what little we know of behavior changes in monkeys, apes, and humans, there is good reason to suspect that there exists a trend toward the retention of juvenile behavioral traits into adulthood in humans. As one such behavior he cited the infantile pattern of clinging characteristic of all the more advanced primates. In humans this is seen in all sorts of contact behavior, and in some cultures in the kind of formalized greeting seen in the *abrazo* of Latins. In monkeys the embrace is somewhat less frequently seen than in apes or humans. Mason draws attention to the prominence of such traits as playfulness, curiosity, and inventiveness in human behavior, the persistence of infantile attachments, and similar traits, and suggests that if it could be shown that behavioral neoteny is a generalized human condition, all such traits would be seen in a different light—as would the loose relationship between hormonal factors and sex and maternal behavior. Mason goes on to inquire, "Could neoteny be one of the reasons it has been so difficult to discover instinctual elements in human behavior, why the great students of human nature have felt compelled to postulate broad, pervasive forces such as the libido and the death wish to explain the instinctual basis of human motivations?''

As a result of the neotenous trends in the organization of behavior in primate evolution, Mason points out, the human infant's needs for social stimulation are less specific than those of the nonhuman primates. The range of equivalent stimuli are wider, development is less dependent on the particular features of stimulation, and the relations to specific forms of stimulus deprivation are more variable and diffuse.

Once a developmental sequence is set in motion, the human infant shows a greater tendency to elaborate on it than the monkey or ape. There is, for example, a progressive enrichment in stereotyped movements from monkey to man. Infant monkeys show little, if any, "spontaneous" sound production. "Chimpanzees 'invent' lip noises, clicking sounds, and the like; but only the human infant truly babbles." This kind of elaboration is seen also in the progressive enrichment and complication of the patterns of playful exploration of objects.

Mason goes on to make the important point that because of the retardation of growth rates and the "loosening" of behavioral organization, developmental stages are less sharply delimited in humans than in other primates, and there is a much stronger tendency for behavior to reflect a blending or intermingling of different developmental stages, different response patterns, and different motivational systems. "Of all primates," Mason adds, "man has gone farthest in an evolutionary venture in which the reliability and efficiency of instinctive patterns have been sacrificed to achieve the behavioral plasticity and the liberation of psychic energy that are so much a part of the human condition.''

David Jonas and Doris Klein

In a book entitled *Man-Child: A Study of the Infantilization of Man*, published in 1970, a husband and wife team, David Jonas (a psychiatrist) and Doris Klein (a writer with some training in anthropology), make use of the data relating to neoteny in a unique way. They see the "infantilization" of humans as a regressive development "moving backwards in terms of his physical endowments while overcompensating for his deficiencies with a hypertrophied neocortex." They perceive behind the facade of humans the nature of the child, a child who is rearranging the environment without regard to the consequences. In every aspect of their lives, the authors maintain, humans are increasingly showing infantile attitudes and responses. "Like Mendeleyev,"* they write, "we were collectors of data, in an attempt to find a correlation between man's prolonged childhood and the widespread prevalence of behavioral and social immaturity on the one hand and possible anatomical and physiological concomitants on the other."

Unfortunately, the authors have completely failed to understand the meaning of neoteny, and for their purposes seem to confuse it with "childishness" or, worse, infantilism. It is, of course, true that were it not for the unique evolution of the human neocortex, humans would not be capable of getting into the troubles they have managed to create for themselves and others on this planet, but to reason that the neocortex is responsible for such behavior is to commit the fallacy of *post hoc, ergo propter hoc* (because one thing follows another, therefore one is the cause of the other). It is not man's neocortex nor his neoteny that is responsible for his difficulties, but the socialized organization and uses to which they have been put. Furthermore, what the authors perceive as infantilized behavior in adolescents and in adults is far from being so, for this is clearly behavior patterned on socially generated models.

For the rest the book is marred by many errors, misattributions, and is otherwise flawed, although it is not altogether without merit.

Robert B. Cairns

Robert B. Cairns, Professor of Psychology at the University of North Carolina, in an article on "The Ontogeny and Phylogeny of Social Interactions," published in 1976, makes the point that not all human social development is neotenous social development. While some features of human behavior fit the neoteny hypothesis, others do not. These include the accelerated use of language and symbolic communication, along with advanced memory storage and recall capabilities. What Cairns fails to understand is that these very features are present as neotenous potentialities in fetus, infant, and child, and therefore fit the neoteny hypothesis perfectly well, as does his suggestion that

---

* Russian physicist, discoverer of the periodic law of the elements.

what has been neotenized in humans has been social and behavioral flexibility.

In broad overview, Cairns argues, both major types of hetero-chronies, neoteny *and* acceleration (the appearance of a mature trait of the ancestor in the youthful stages of the descendant), appear to be involved in the multiple differences between human and related primate forms. Cairns, quite rightly, emphasizes that multiple behavior differences may be influenced by a modest shift in the timing of physiological development, and cites good evidence in support of that statement.

Roderic Gorney

Roderic Gorney, Assistant Clinical Professor of Psychiatry at the University of California at Los Angeles, in his book *The Human Agenda* (1972) devotes many pages to the demonstration of how it has come about that humans owe their neoteny to the enormous scope of their adaptive capacities. At the same time, he points out, the individual, during his lifetime, usually goes through a process of specialization, which gradually narrows the range of choices his basic neoteny has rendered open to him. The more specialized we become, the more we miss the omnipotentialities of youth.

Gorney sees the temporary imbalance of development, which has allowed humans to become their only real enemies, as correctable through the neoteny of the mind. The instruments of repair are the dilating imagination and loving playfulness, "qualities of the young mammal taken over, and expanded by the neotenic human mind."

R. Dale Guthrie

In his fascinating book *Body Hot Spots: The Anatomy of Human Social Organs and Behavior* (1976), R. Dale Guthrie, Professor of Biology at the University of Alaska, has devoted an excellent chapter to a discussion of the role neoteny has played in the development of both physical and behavioral traits in humans. Among his many original observations Guthrie points out that under primitive conditions a certain conservatism, a reliance on the tested, tends to be customary. A child, however, has little to lose from exploratory failure and much to gain from success. For the adult the price of change may be more severe.

Guthrie suggests that children must have been the great innovators of early human lifestyles. Children had greater leisure and social freedom to experiment with new ways of doing things, with trying different ways of modifying tools, with making pets of the young of wild animals, with the making of music, and so on. "Somewhere along the line," writes Guthrie, "it became increasingly advantageous to continue the child's enthusiasm for new experiences on into adult life." Perhaps, says Guthrie, our childhood behavior is extended into adulthood. Common signals of appeasement, such as childlike or youthful behavior, higher pitched voice, diminished height, and the like, are examples of social neoteny. From appeasement gestures those of friendship are derived; we establish deeper friendships and we are more social than other animals.

Even our faces have retained a more childlike appearance, and thus a less threatening or intimidating visage. Smooth skin texture would appear to be another example of social neoteny. In adult apes the skin is rough, but it is fairly smooth in the young.

Guthrie sees as socially neotenic the pink cheek spot, associated with youth and vigor, which is made up for with rouge by women who lack it naturally; elongated eyelashes—eyeliner pencils or brushes are employed to make the eyes appear disproportionately large for the face, in imitation of the eyes of the child; the exaggerated everted lip of the lipstick ad model, which transmits an effective neotenic signal, the "bigger-than-life baby." As Guthrie points out, any time adults profit from looking like a child—that is, by eliciting care and protection from adults—adults will mimic such traits. Women and girls profited from looking more childlike than men. For the moment the adult becomes a child to be comforted, and cared for.

Stephen Jay Gould

The most important discussion of neoteny to have appeared in recent years in Stephen Jay Gould's book *Ontogeny and Phylogeny* (1977). Gould is Professor of Geology at Harvard University; his main interest is vertebrate paleontology. In his very readable book, Gould is concerned to throw some light on the relationship between individual development (ontogeny) and the evolution of species and lineages (phylogeny). In well-reasoned and solidly based ordering and examination of the evidence, Gould shows how gene regulation produces changes in the relative time of appearance and rate of development of traits already present in ancestral, fetal, or juvenile forms; that is, by heterochrony or the displacement of traits in time. The primary evolutionary value of heterochrony appears to lie in the immediate ecological or environmental advantages it offers for slow or rapid maturation, rather than in the long-term changes in form that are generally postulated.

"Neoteny," Gould declares early in the first chapter of his book, "has been a (probably *the*) major determinant of human evolution. . . . Human development has slowed down. Within this 'matrix of retardation,' adaptive features of ancestral juveniles are easily retained. Retardation as a life-history strategy for longer learning and socialization may be far more important in human evolution than any of its morphological consequences." These words constitute the essence of the fifty-two pages of Gould's penultimate chapter on the role played by retardation, by neoteny, in human evolution. It is a brilliant chapter, and for our purposes, constitutes by far the best support for the role and reality of neoteny or paedomorphosis as a factor in human evolution since de Beer's *Ancestors and Embryos* (1940).

However, unlike virtually all other workers who have discussed neoteny in relation to human evolution, Gould has noted that much of human evolution has occurred not merely as a result of developmental retardation at various stages of ancestral and fetal development; he drew attention to the fact that such retardation has also occurred at various juvenile stages of the species to which we belong. In an admirable article entitled "The Child as Man's Real Father" (1975), and in his book, Gould argues that the best evidence of human neoteny is that as adults we resemble our own fetal and juvenile stages. It is indeed a fact that retention of their own species-specific and subspecific juvenile traits has played a highly significant role in the evolution of humans. I showed in 1960 that such juvenilization or paedomorphosis has proceeded further, morphologically at least, in Mongoloid peoples than in Caucasoids and Negroids. In some Negroids, however, such as the extinct Boskopoids of Africa of about 100,000 years ago, paedormorphic traits, among them the very large brain of 1,700 cubic centimeters (as compared with 1,400 cc of contemporary humans), as well as a vertical-faced profile, and a height of about five feet six inches, had developed further and earlier than in any other variety of humankind. Some of these traits are preserved in what are believed to be their descendants, the present-day gatherer-hunters known as the Khoi San or Bushmen of South Africa.

Conclusion

Our survey of the history of the development of the concept of neoteny or paedomorphism has by no means been exhaustive. Some discussions of interest have been omitted. All of them agree in recognizing that neoteny has been an important factor in the evolution of humankind. All of them either explicitly or implicitly recognize that in development from conception to terminal age the organism is changing continuously. The genes regulating development interact with the environment to synthesize the substances that result in the differentiation of the various tissues and organs. This differentiation is under the control of genes that exert their effects by varying the rates at which chemical reactions occur. What this means is that individuals can vary in the amount of development they have undergone. Some are more grown up than others. Natural selection acts upon variations along the full time-scale of development. As de Beer put it, "All stages of the life-history are available for the selection of those forms most efficiently adapted to their environments, and these will not always be the forms of the adult ancestor." The evolutionary history of many groups is characterized by delayed development, prolongation of the youthful stages into the phase of sexual maturity, and the discarding of the old adult stage. In such cases the adult stage of the descendant resembles the youthful stage of the ancestor. This mode of evolution, called neoteny or paedomorphosis, has been followed by the most successful groups of animals, from a variety of ammonites, through insects and other forms, to humans. In humans it is especially clear that this process involves the retention of many of the individual's own juvenile traits into adult life.

Not all human traits are neotenous, nor are all neotenous changes brought about by the slowing-down of development. The outstanding example of a non-neotenous rate of development in humans is the growth of the lower extremities, which are considerably longer than in any other primate. The best example of a neotenous change brought about by the acceleration of the rate of development is the human brain, which continues to grow into early adult life.

We conclude, then, that it seems indisputable that the morphological as well as the behavioral potentialities that make us specifically human are the result principally of neoteny or paedomorphosis.

Appendix B

GLOSSARY

Acceleration. A speeding up of development so that a feature appears earlier in the individual descendant than it did in an ancestor.

Adaptation. A trait of the organism that, in the environment it inhabits, improves its chances of leaving descendants.

Adaptive radiation. Evolution, from a primitive type of organism, or from a basically successful adaptation, of divergent forms adapted to distinct modes of life.

Adduction. To pull a part of the body toward the median axis.

Aggression. A term difficult to define because there are many forms of aggressive behavior. A working definition as good as any is the actual or intended imposition of an individual's or group's wishes on others against their will.

Allele. One of the two forms of a gene.

Allometry. The study and measurement of the relative growth of a part of an organism in comparison with the whole.

Altricial. In which the young are born in large litters after short gestation periods, helplessness, and rapid development.

Anabolism. The process by which food is changed into living tissue.

Anatomy. The study of the structure of a body or organism.

Anlage. The basis of a later development of a structure.

Anovulatory. Without ovulation.

Anthropoid. Manlike. Referring to the manlike apes—the orangutan, chimpanzee, gorilla, and sometimes the gibbon.

Apes. Members of the family Pongidae, consisting of the gibbons, orangutan, chimpanzee, and gorilla.

Apocrine glands. A type of sweat gland in which part of its apex is cast off together with its secretory products.

Arboreal. Adapted for living in trees.

Australopithecine. A member of the African hominid forms of several million years ago.

Australopithecus africanus. A manlike South African species.

Bacteriocidal. A substance that kills bacteria.

Bacteriostatic. A substance that prevents the multiplication of bacteria.

Biogenetic Law. Ernst Haeckel's term for his theory that in individual development the organism climbs, as it were, its own family tree—ontogeny recapitulates phylogeny.

Brachycephaly. Broad-headness.

Buccal. Toward the cheek side.

Canine teeth. The eyeteeth.

Caucasoid. A large major group of humankind, including the peoples of Europe, North Africa, the Near East, India, etc.

Cephalic index. A measure of the human head computed by dividing its maximum breadth by its maximum length and multiplying by a hundred.

Chromosome. One of a number of double-thread-shaped bodies possibly made of protein, situated in the nucleus of the cell and carrying the genes. A code center.

Clandestine evolution. Evolutionary change that takes place in the young phases of development while the adult modifications, if any, are minor. If neoteny then occurs, the phylogeny will undergo an abrupt modification and start off in an altogether new direction. The young or early modified forms will show no transitional evolutionary traits between themselves and their adult ancestors. Thus, there will be a "gap" between such forms and their ancestors. This explains the gaps that exists in the fossil record between most forms.

Colostrum. The lemony-yellowish fluid, rich in protein and immunity-conferring substances, secreted by the breast some days before and after the birth of young.

Conceptus. The organism from conception to birth.

Conjunctiva. The mucous membrane lining the inner surface of the eyelids and covering the front part of the eyeball.

Convolution. Surface fold of the brain.

Cranial capacity. The volume of the brain-bearing part of the skull.

Cranium. The skull minus the lower jaw.

Culture. The part of the environment that is learned. The human-made part of the environment.

Deciduous. Referring to the milk teeth.

Development. Increase in complexity.

Diastema. The gap between two adjacent teeth.

Dolichocephaly. Long-headedness.

Eccrine glands. The common sweat glands that secrete the clear watery sweat, important in heat regulation.

Ecology. The study of the interactions between organisms and their environment.

Embryo. The human organism up to the third month.

Embryology. The study of the formation and development of embryos.

Endocrine. Referring to the glands of internal secretion.

Environment. The conditions acting upon the organism—internal as well as external.

Epicanthic fold. A fold of skin from the upper eyelid that covers the inner angle of the eye.

Epigamic. Relating to the mating of animals and the characteristics of color, etc., that serve to attract the opposite sex during courtship.

Epithelium. One or more layers of cellular tissue covering surfaces, forming glands, and lining most cavities of the body.

Evolution. Development, by descent, with modification.

Exterogestation. The exterior gestation the infant spends outside the womb, until he begins to crawl around under his own steam.

Family. A classificatory category (taxon) consisting of a number of similar genera. The name of a family ends in *-idae.*

Fetalization. Bolk's term for neoteny or paedomorphosis, but with emphasis on the retention of fetal traits.

Fetus. In humans the organism from the commencement of the third month of gestation to birth.

Fontéchevade. Fragmentary portions of two fossil skulls found in southwestern France, probably belonging to the first interglacial.

Foramen magnum. The large opening at the base of the skull through which the spinal cord passes.

Fossil. Remains of an organism, or direct evidence of its presence, preserved in rocks.

Gene. The physical unit of heredity, a small region in a chromosome consisting mainly of DNA (deoxyribonucleic acid).

Genetic Drift or the Sewall Wright Effect. The nonselective or random distribution or extinction or fixation of genes in a population.

Genome. The sum total of the genes of an organism.

Genotype. Same as genome, used in contrast to phenotype (*q.v.*).

Genus. The main subdivision of a Family, made up of a number of closely related species.

Gerontomorphosis. Evolution by means of modification of adult traits.

Gonad. The organ in animals that produces reproductive cells.

Growth. Increase in size or amplitude.

Gyrus. Same as *convolution* (*q.v.*). A fold of the gray matter of the brain between fissures.

Heterochrony. An evolutionary change in the timing of development affecting the rate of development or the appearance of a feature in a descendant form.

Hirsute. Hairy.

Hominid. A member of the Family Hominidae.

Hominidae. The Family of all species of humankind, including the australopithecines.

Hominization. The process of change to humankind.

Homo erectus. Formerly *Pithecanthropus erectus;* Middle Pleistocene form of human.

Homo sapiens. The living species of the genus *Homo,* as well as some extinct forms of the species.

Human. Belonging to or typical of women and men, children, and the conceptus.

Hypermorphosis. Additional development where evolution has resulted in progressive increase in size, or where maturity is delayed relatively to body-characters. The long legs of humans are an example. The lengthening of the legs of humans must have occurred during the evolution of humans from anthropoids whose legs were shorter.

Intelligence. The ability to make the most appropriately successful response to the particular challenge of the situation.

Interactional synchrony. Harmonic interaction between two or more persons.

Labial. Pertaining to or toward the lips.

Lacrimal gland. The gland above the eye that secretes tears.

Larva. The early, free-living, immature form of any animal that changes structurally when it becomes an adult.

Libido. The sexual urge or psychic energy generally.

Lysozyme. A bacteriocidal and bacteriostatic substance secreted by many of the membranes of the body.

Malocclusion. Abnormal relation of upper and lower teeth.

Mammal. Member of a class of animals characterized by hair, milk secretion, diaphragm used in respiration, lower jaw made up of a single pair of bones, presence of only left systemic arch, and three auditory ossicles in each middle ear connecting eardrum and inner ear.

Mandible. The lower jaw.

Maturity. Being fully grown or developed.

Maxilla. The upper jaw.

Melanin. A complex, dark brown pigment, which in various concentrations affects the color of the skin, hair, and eyes.

Menarche. The first menstruation.

Metamorphosis. A change in form, structure or function as a result of development.

Microcephaly. Abnormally small head, associated with mental retardation.

Monotocous. Having one offspring at a birth.

Morphology. The study of form, usually involving the study of the relation between function, structure, and form.

Mosaic evolution. The fact that there is an unequal evolution of the structures of an organism. One structure may be under particularly heavy selection pressure, while others lag behind. For example, in humans the erect posture preceded the development of the large brain. Like a mosaic made up of different bits and pieces and colors, so the parts of an organism are made up of different parts that have evolved at different rates.

Mutation. A change in the structure of a gene resulting in a transmissible hereditary modification in the expression of a trait.

Mutation pressure. The measure of the action of mutations in tending to alter the frequency of a gene in a given population.

Myelinization. The deposition of the white fatty sheath about certain nerve fibers.

Nasolacrimal duct. The duct draining the eye fluids into the nasal cavity.

Natural selection. Differential fertility. The fact that organisms that possess a trait or traits that enable them to adapt better to the environment than organisms that lack such a trait or traits are more likely to leave a larger progeny. Darwin, who originally suggested the principle, described it as follows: "As many more individuals of each species are born than can possibly survive, and as, consequently, there is a frequently recurring struggle for existence, it follows that any being, if it vary however slightly in any manner profitable to itself, under the complex and sometimes varying conditions of life, will have a better chance of surviving, and thus be *naturally selected*. From the strong principle of inheritance, any selected variety will tend to propagate its new and modified form." (Charles Darwin, *The Origin of Species*, 1859.)

Neandertal man. Humans of Mousterian culture of the Upper Pleistocene prior to the reduction of the face and teeth of the Middle Pleistocene.

Neonate. The human infant from birth to the end of the second week.

Neoteny. The retention of fetal or juvenile traits by retardation of developmental processes. Same as *Paedomorphosis* (*q.v.*).

Nubility. The age at which, on average, the human female becomes capable of conceiving and carrying a fetus to term (between seventeen and twenty-two years).

Occipital condyles. The rounded processes on each side of the foramen magnum that rest the skull on the vertebral column.

Ontogeny. The life-cycle of the organism, especially during individual development.

Orthognathy. The nonprojection of the jaws in front of the cranium.

Oxytocin. A pituitary gland hormone that stimulates the tubules of the breast, induces the "letdown reflex" (which causes the milk to flow freely from the breast), induces massive contractions of the uterus, and assists in maternalizing the mother's behavior.

Paedomorphosis. The retention of fetal or juvenile traits by retardation of developmental processes.

Paleolithic. "The Old Stone Age," comprising the early, middle, and upper age of stone toolmaking.

Phenotype. The manifest traits of the organism; the product of the joint interaction of environment with genotype.

Phylogeny. The evolutionary lines of descent or development of any species.

Pithecanthropines. General name for the members of *Homo erectus.*

Pithecoid. Apelike.

Polytocous. Giving birth to more than one offspring.

Postpartum. The period following childbirth.

Precocial. In which the young are born in small litters, are relatively well developed, and are mobile shortly after birth.

Premaxillary suture. The suture separating the maxillary from the pre-maxillary bone on the facial aspect of the skull.

Progenesis. Paedomorphosis produced by precocious sexual matura-tion of a morphologically juvenile organism.

Prolactin. One of the hormones that stimulates and sustains lactation, and also serves to maternalize maternal behavior.

Promine. A hormone-like substance secreted by the thymus gland, thought to be a "Peter Pan" hormone.

Recapitulation. Passing through ancestral adult stages in embryonic and juvenile development of descendants.

Reflex. An automatic reaction to a stimulus.

Regulatory genes. Genes regulating development by turning on or off structural genes that produce proteins for the construction of body parts.

Retardation. A slowing-down of development so that a feature or trait appears later in a descendant than it did in an ancestor.

Ritualization. The modification of a behavior pattern to serve a com-municative function.

Selection. The maintenance of certain genotypes having adaptive value in contrast with others that do not, and that therefore are unlikely to do as well by way of leaving a progeny.

Selection pressure. The measure of the action of selection in tending to alter the frequency of a gene in a population.

Selective advantage. The genotypic condition of an organism or group of organisms that increases its chances, relative to others, of rep-resentation in later generations.

Sexual selection. Conscious selection on the basis of some preferred sexual trait as a factor of evolution.

Skull. The bony framework of the head, composed of the cranial bones and the bones of the face.

Somatic. Relating to the body.

Specialization. Development of special adaptations to a particular habitat or mode of life, resulting in divergence of traits from an-cestral forms.

Species. A group of actually or potentially interbreeding natural popu-lations, which is more or less reproductively isolated from other such populations.

Supraorbital tori. Overhanging eyebrow ridges.

Suture. The edges at which the different bones of the skull come together, and with age mostly unite.

Symbiosis. The intimate living together of two kinds of organisms; also, a similar relationship of interdependence between persons or groups.

Synostosis. Union of adjacent cranial bones at sutural junctions.

Uterogestation. Gestation within the womb.

References
and Notes

INTRODUCTION

Page and line

5:24–36   Philippe Ariès, *Centuries of Childhood*. New York: Alfred A. Knopf, 1962.

5:36–38   A remark attributed to the headmaster of Charterhouse School in England, in the 1920s

6:32 to   Julius Kollmann, "Das Uberwintern von europäischen Frosch-
7:1   und die Umwandlung des mexikanischen axolotl," *Verhandlungen der naturforschenden Gesellschaft*, Basel, vol. 7, 1884, pp. 387–398.

6:36–37   At Freiberg University in 1865. See E. G. Boulenger, "Class Batrachia (or Amphibia)," in *Natural History*, Charles Tate Regan (ed.). New York: Hillman-Curl, 1937, p. 301.

7:3–10   Havelock Ellis, *Man and Woman*. London: Walter Scott Publishing Co., 1894, p. 25.

:11–24   Louis Bolk, *Das Problem der Menschwerdung*. Jena: Gustav Fischer, 1926.

:25–36   J. B. S. Haldane, *The Causes of Evolution*. London: Longmans, 1932, p. 150.

:37 to   Konrad Lorenz, "Part and Parcel in Animal and Human Soci-
8:8   eties" (1950), in *Studies in Animal and Human Behavior*, vol. 2, pp. 115–195. Cambridge: Harvard University Press, 1971.

:7   Arnold Gehlen, *Der Mensch: Seine Natur und Seine Stellung in der Welt*. Wiesbaden: Athenaion, 1940/1976. English translation in preparation.

:8 to   Stephen Jay Gould, *Ontogeny and Phylogeny*. Cambridge: Har-
9:7   vard University Press, 1977.

15:1–13   Adrienne L. Zihlman, John E. Cronin, Douglas L. Cramer, and Vincent M. Sarich, "Pygmy Chimpanzee as a Possible Pro-

Page and line

totype for the Common Ancestor of Humans, Chimpanzees and Gorillas," *Nature,* vol. 275, 1978, pp. 744–745.

15:14–24　Laura Manuelidis and John C. Wu, "Homology between Human and Simian Repeated DNA," *Nature,* 1978, pp. 92–94; Elizabeth J. Bruce, and Francisco J. Ayala, "Humans and Apes Are Genetically Very Similar," *Nature,* vol. 276, 1978, pp. 264–265.

:28–31　Julian S. Huxley, *Problems of Relative Growth.* New York: Lincoln MacVeagh, 1932, p.239.

:31–33　Julian S. Huxley, *Evolution: The Modern Synthesis.* New York and London: Harper & Brothers, 1942, p. 532.

1. NEOTENY AND THE
BIOLOGICAL EVOLUTION
OF HUMANKIND

16:4–8　Arthur Keith, *A New Theory of Human Evolution.* London: Watts & Co., 1948, p. 195.

25:6–7　Gavin de Beer, *Embryos and Ancestors.* 3rd ed. New York: Oxford University Press, 1958, p. 70.

26:11–16　Franz Weidenreich, "Morphology of Solo Man," in *Anthropological Papers of the American Museum of Natural History,* vol. 43, 1951, pp. 205–290.

:16–30　Ashley Montagu, "Natural Selection and the Form of the Breast in the Human Female," *Journal of the American Medical Association,* vol. 180, 1961, pp. 108–109; Ashley Montagu, "Breastfeeding and Its Relation to Morphological, Behavioral, and Psychological Development." In *Breastfeeding and Food Policy in a Hungry World,* Dana Raphael (ed.). New York: Academic Press, 1979, pp. 189–197.

:36 to
27:1–2　Cathleen B. Clark, "A Preliminary Report on Weaning among Chimpanzees of the Gombe National Park, Tanzania," *Primate Bio-Social Development: Biological, Social, and Ecological Determinants.* New York: Garland Publishing Co., 1977, pp. 235–260.

28:9–11　Louis Bolk, "The Problem of Orthognathism," *Proc. Section Sciences Kon. Akad. Wetens. Amsterdam,* vol. 25, 1923, pp. 371–380.

29:12–14　E. V. Glanville, "Nasal Shape, Prognathism and Adaptation in Man," *American Journal of Physical Anthropology,* vol. 30, 1969, pp. 29–37.

:23–28　Aidan Macfarlane, *The Psychology of Childbirth.* Cambridge: Harvard University Press, 1977.

Page and line

29:28–38   R. H. Wright, *The Science of Smell*. New York: Basic Books, 1964, pp. 43–56.

31:12–15   Robert Yerkes and Ada W. Yerkes, *The Great Apes*. New Haven: Yale University Press, 1929, pp. 161, 255, 299.

:16 to / 33:27   Ashley Montagu, "Natural Selection and the Origin and Evolution of Weeping in Man," *Science,* vol. 130, 1959, pp. 1572–1573; Ashley Montagu, "Natural Selection and the Origin and Evolution of Weeping in Man," *Journal of the American Medical Association,* vol. 174, 1960, pp. 392–398.

32:10–19   T. H. Holmes et al., *The Nose: Experimental Study of Reactions within the Nose during Varying Life Experiences*. Springfield, Illinois: C C Thomas, 1950; A. W. Proetz, *Displacement Method of Sinus Diagnosis and Treatment,* 2nd. ed., St. Louis: Annals Publishing Co., 1946.

:20–25   F. Ridley, "Antibacterial Body Present in Great Concentration in Tears, and Its Relation to Infection of Human Eye," *Proceedings of the Royal Society of Medicine (Section on Ophthalmology),* vol. 21, 1928, pp. 55–56.

31:16 to / 32:9   Ashley Montagu, Reference, vide supra.

33:39 to / 34:2   R. Dale Guthrie, *Body Hot Spots*. New York: Van Nostrand Reinhold Co., 1976, p. 164.

:8–13   A. R. Radcliffe-Brown, *The Andaman Islanders*. Cambridge (England): At the University Press, 1933, p. 117.

35:12–24   Ashley Montagu, *Touching: The Human Significance of the Skin*. 2nd. ed. New York: Harper & Row, 1978.

36:28–32   Donald G. Paterson, *Physique and Intellect*. New York: Century Company, 1930.

37:3–6   R. Dale Guthrie, op. cit., p. 163.

37:17–18   Stephen Jay Gould, "Mickey Mouse Meets Konrad Lorenz," *Natural History,* vol. 88, 1979, pp. 30–36.

:19–24   R. Dale Guthrie, op. cit., p. 163.

39:20–36   John Hurrell Crook, "Sexual Selection, Dimorphism, and Social Organization in the Primates," In *Sexual Selection and the Descent of Man, 1871–1971*. Bernard Campbell (ed.). Chicago: Aldine Publishing Co., 1972, pp. 273–274.

40:16–22   James Couper Brash, *The Aetiology of Irregularity and Malocclusion of the Teeth*. 2nd ed. London: The Dental Board of the United Kingdom, 1956, p. 292.

:33 to / 41:1–8   Ashley Montagu, "The Premaxilla in the Primates," *Quarterly Review of Biology,* vol. 10, 1935, pp. 32–59, 181–208.

44:16–36   Ashley Montagu, *The Reproductive Development of the Female*. 3rd. ed. Littleton, Mass: PSG Publishing Co., 1979.

:16–36   Ibid.

:36 to / 45:1–7   Ashley Montagu: *Touching: The Human Significance of the Skin*. 2nd ed. New York: Harper & Row, 1978.

Page and line

45:38 to   Gavin de Beer. *Embryos and Ancestors.* 3rd ed. London and
46:1–10   New York: Oxford University Press, 1958, pp. 36, 113.
:13 to   Louis Bolk, "Origin of Racial Characteristics in Man," *Amer-*
53:1–39   *ican Journal of Physical Anthropology,* vol. 13, 1929, pp.
           1–28.
46:1–10   Richard C. Lewontin, "Adaptation," *Scientific American,* vol.
           239, 1978, pp. 212–230.
:28 to   Arthur Keith, "The Differentiation of Mankind into Racial
47:1–10   Types," *Report of the 87th Meeting of the British Associa-*
           tion for the Advancement of Sciences, London, 1919,
           pp. 275–281: W. Pfuhl, "The Relation between Racial and
           Constitutional Investigations," *Zeitschrift für Konstitu-*
           tionslehre, vol. 9, 1923, pp. 172–196: Louis Bolk, loc. cit.,
           p. 4.
:19–22   Louis Berman, *The Glands Regulating Personality.* New York:
           W. W. Norton, 1921, and many editions thereafter.
:22–24   Charles Stockard, "Human Types and Growth Reactions," *The*
           American Journal of Anatomy, vol. 31, 1923, pp. 261–288.
:24–26   Charles Stockard, *The Physical Basis of Personality.* New York:
           W. W. Norton, 1931.
:27–28   Charles Stockard, *The Genetic and Endocrine Basis for Differ-*
           ences in Form and Behavior. Philadelphia: The Wistar Insti-
           tute, 1941.
:28–38   Louis Bolk, loc. cit., 5.
:39 to   Joseph Shellshear, "The Thymus Gland in the Chinese," *China*
48:1–7   *Medical Journal,* vol. 38, 1924, pp. 646–657.
:8–18   Albert Szent-Györgi, *Bioenergetics.* New York: Academic
           Press, 1957, p. 143; Albert Szent-Györgi, "Growth and Or-
           ganization," *Biochemical Journal,* vol. 98, 1966, pp. 641–
           644.
:19–23   Victor A. Najjar, "The Mechanism of Antibody-Antigen Reac-
           tion and the Physiological Function of γ-globulin," In *A*
           Symposium on the Child, John Askin et al., eds. Baltimore:
           The Johns Hopkins Press, 1967, pp. 208–232.
:23–32   T. D. Luckey, (ed.), *Thymic Hormones.* Baltimore: University
           Park Press, 1973; A. Hegyeli and J. McLaughlin, "Constit-
           uents of the Thymus Gland and Their Relation to Growth,
           Fertility, Muscle, and Cancer," *Proceedings of the Na-*
           tional Academy of Sciences, vol. 48, 1962, pp. 1439–1442.
:38 to   Louis Bolk, op. cit., p. 6.
50:1–3   Ashley Montagu, *The Reproductive Development of the Female.*
:11–17   3d ed., Littleton, Mass.: PSG Publishing Co., 1979.
:17–24   P. K. Ito, "Comparative Biometrical Study of Physique of
           Japanese Women Born and Reared under Different Envi-
           ronments," *Human Biology,* vol. 14, 1942, pp. 279–351.
51:17–23   Franz Weidenreich, "The Brachycephalization of Recent Man-

Page and line

kind," *Southwestern Journal of Anthropology,* vol. 1, 1945, pp. 1–54.

51:30–40   Ashley Montagu, "The Premaxilla in Man," *Journal of the American Dental Association,* vol. 23, 1936, pp. 2043–2057; Ashley Montagu, "The Significance of the Variability of the Upper Lateral Incisor Teeth in Man," *Human Biology,* vol. 12, 1940, pp. 323–358.

52:1 to   Louis Bolk, op. cit., p. 27.
53:1–39

52:34 to   C. U. Ariens Kappers, "Indices for the Anthropology of the
53:1–5   Brain Applied to Chinese Dolicho- and Brachycephalic Foetuses and Neonati," *Proc. Kon. Akad. Wetensch. Amsterdam,* vol. 30, 1927, pp. 81–94.

:14–27   Louis Bolk, op. cit., p. 18.

:31–39   Theodosius Dobzhansky and Ashley Montagu, "Natural Selection and the Mental Capacities of Mankind," *Science,* vol. 105, 1947, pp. 587–590.

54:1 to   Ashley Montagu, "Breastfeeding and Its Relation to Mor-
55:1–13   phological, Behavioral, and Psychological Development." In *Breastfeeding and Food Policy in a Hungry World,* Dana Raphael (ed.). New York: Academic Press, 1979, pp. 189–197.

54:30–33   William Painter, *The Palace of Pleasure.* London: Tottell and Jones, 1566, I, 63.

:33 to   Ashley Montagu, *Touching: The Human Significance of the Skin.*
55:1–13   2nd ed. New York: Harper & Row, 1978; Ashley Montagu, "Mother's Touch," *Science Digest,* vol. 89. 1981, p. 16.

57:2–8   Yas Kuno, *Human Perspiration.* Springfield, Illinois: C C
:8–10   Thomas, 1956.

   Yas Kuno, loc. cit., p. 341.

:1–26   C. Loring Brace and Ashley Montagu, *Human Evolution.* 2nd ed. New York: The Macmillan Company, 1977, pp. 312–314.

55:18 to   Richard B. Lee and Irven DeVore (eds.), *Man the Hunter.*
56:1–8   Chicago: Aldine Publishing Co., 1968.

55:18 to   C. S. Coon, S. M. Garn, and J. B. Birdsell, *Races.* Springfield,
56:1–8   Illinois: C C Thomas, 1950, pp. 71–72; S. M. Garn, "Types and Distribution of the Hair in Man," *Annals of the New York Academy of Sciences,* vol. 53, 1951, pp. 498–527.

57:27–32   J. B. Hamilton, "Patterned Loss of Hair in Man: Types and Incidence," *Annals of the New York Academy of Sciences,* vol. 53, 1951, pp. 708–728.

58:1–10   Desmond Morris, *The Naked Ape.* New York: McGraw-Hill, 1967, p. 46.

:19–28   T. T. McConaill and F. L. Ralphs, "Postnatal Development of Hair and Eye Colour with Special Reference to Some

Page and line

Ethnological Problems," *Annals of Eugenics,* vol. 7, 1937,
pp. 218–225.

58:38 to   J. B. Hamilton, Reference 55.
59:1–3

:16–24   Grafton Elliot Smith, *The Evolution of Man.* 2nd ed. London:
Oxford University Press, 1927, p. 66.

:25 to   Ibid., p. 50.
60:1–4

:11–15   Brace and Montagu, op. cit.

:16 to   Ernst Mayr, *Animal Species and Evolution.* Cambridge: Har-
61:1–20   vard University Press, 1963, p. 636.

60:21–32   Adrienne L. Zihlman, John E. Cronin, Douglas L. Cramer, and
Vincent M. Sarich, "Pygmy Chimpanzee as a Possible Pro-
totype for the Common Ancestor of Humans, Chimpanzees, and Gorillas," *Nature,* vol. 275, 1978, pp. 744–746.

61:22–23   Stephen Jay Gould, *Ontogeny and Phylogeny,* Cambridge: Harvard University Press, p. 365 sq.

2. NEOTENY AND THE EVOLUTION OF HUMAN BEHAVIOR

62:1–4   William A. Mason, "Early Social Deprivation in the Nonhuman
Primates: Implications for Human Behavior," in *Environ-
mental Influences,* David C. Glass (ed.), New York:
Rockefeller University Press, 1968, p. 96.

63:32–39   Ralph W. Gerard, "Brains and Behavior," in *The Evolution of
Man's Capacity for Culture,* J. N. Spuhler (ed.), Detroit:
Wayne State University Press, 1959, p. 17.

65:11–15   John Dobbing and Jean Sands, "Timing of Neuroblast Multiplication in Developing Human Brain," *Nature,* vol. 226,
1970, pp. 639–640.

:32–38   Arthur Keith, "Foetalization as a Factor in Human Evolution,"
in Keith's *A New Theory of Human Evolution.* London:
Watts & Co., 1948, p. 199.

67:38–40   D. K. Spelt, "The Conditioning of the Human Fetus *in utero,"
Journal of Experimental Psychology,* vol. 38, 1948, pp.
338–346.

68:32–36   Gaston Viaud, *Intelligence: Its Evolution and Forms.* New York:
Harper & Brothers, 1960.

:68 to   Daniel S. Lehrman, "A Critique of Lorenz's Theory of Instinc-
69:1–2   tive Behavior," *Quarterly Review of Biology,* vol. 28, 1953,
pp. 337–363; *Development and Evolution of Behavior,* Lester R. Aronson et al. (eds.), San Francisco: W. H. Freeman
& Co., 1970; E. Tobach et al. (eds.), *The Biopsychology of
Development.* New York: Academic Press, 1971; R. E.
Passingham, "Changes in the Size and Organization of the

Page and line

Brain in Man and His Ancestors," *Brain, Behavior and Evolution,* vol. 11, 1975, pp. 73–90.

69:2–6   R. E. Passingham. "The Brain and Intelligence," *Brain, Behavior and Evolution,* vol. 11, 1975, pp. 1–15.

69:10–12   Page Smith, *John Adams.* New York: McGraw-Hill, 1962, vol. 1, p. 230.

70:1–9   Ralph S. Solecki, *Shanidar: The First Flower People.* New York: Alfred A. Knopf, 1971.

:9–10   Lucien C. Cuénot, quoted in F.-M. Bergounioux and Joseph Goetz, *Primitive and Prehistoric Religions.* New York: Hawthorn Books, 1966, p. 46.

:11–15   Paul Radin, *Primitive Man as Philosopher.* New York: D. Appleton & Co., 1927.

72:1–4   Aristotle, *Politics.* For the best edition see Ernest Barker, *The Politics of Aristotle.* Oxford: the Clarendon Press, 1946.

:5–9   Ronald A. Fisher, *The Genetical Theory of Natural Selection.* Oxford: the Clarendon Press, 1930.

75:38 to   Ashley Montagu, "Toolmaking, Hunting, and the Origin of
76:1–2   Language," In *Origins and Evolution of Language and Speech,* Stevan Harnad, Horst D. Steklis, and Jane Lancaster (eds.), Annals of the New York Academy of Sciences, vol. 280, 1976 pp. 266–274.

77:30–35   Hermann J. Muller, "Progress and Prospects in Human Genetics," *American Journal of Human Genetics,* vol. 1, 1949, pp. 1–18.

:38 to   Ashley Montagu, *Man's Most Dangerous Myth: The Fallacy of*
78:1–10   *Race.* 5th ed. New York: Oxford University Press, 1974.

:14–32   William Kingdon Clifford, "On Some of the Conditions of Mental Development," in *Lectures and Essays,* London: Macmillan & Company, 1886, pp. 71–72.

3. WHY ARE HUMANS BORN SO HELPLESS AND WHY DO THEY REMAIN SO LONG IMMATURE?

79:1–9   Lucretius, *On the Nature of Things,* Book V, Section 1, Lines 220–230. *De Rerum Natura,* Translated by R. C. Trevelyan, Cambridge: the University Press, 1937, p. 185.

80:8–21   Nicholas Murray Butler, "Anaximander on the Prolongation of Infancy in Man," in *Classical Studies in Honour of Henry Drisler,* New York: Macmillan & Company, 1894, pp. 8–10; Charles R. Eastman, "Anaximander, Earliest Precursor of Darwin," *Popular Science Monthly,* vol. 67, 1905, pp. 701–706; Anita Schosch, *Images of Childhood.* New York: Mayflower Books, 1978; Bernard Wishy, *The Child and the Republic.* Philadelphia: University of Pennsylvania Press, 1968.

80:22 to   Lucretius, *op. cit.* Book V, lines 1019–1028.
81:1–6

Page and line

81:38 to   John Fiske, *Outlines of Cosmic Philosophy, Based on the Doc-*
82:1–12   *trine of Evolution*. London: the Macmillan Company, 1874.

82:13–29   E. H. Russell, "Introduction," in Ella Haskell, *Child Observa-tions*. Boston, p. xix, 1896.

83:32–36   Z. Litvai, "Die Anatomischen und Biologischen Eigenschaften des Nervensystems bei Neugeborenen," *Annales Pedait-rici,* vol. 174, 1950, pp. 252–274.

:36 to   E. H. Watson and G. H. Lowrey, *Growth and Development of*
84:1–9   *Children*. Chicago: Year Book Medical Publishers, 1967; Frank Falkner and J. M. Tanner (eds.), *Human Growth.* New York and London: Plenum Press, 1978; John A. Davis and John Dobbing (eds.), *Scientific Foundations of Paediat-rics*. Philadelphia: W. B. Saunders, 1974.

86:4–5   Weston La Barre, *The Human Animal*. Chicago: University of Chicago Press, 1954.

87:16–32   J. Z. Young, *An Introduction to the Study of Man*. Oxford: the Clarendon Press, 1971, p. 479.

:22–26   Ashley Montagu (ed.), *Man and Aggression*. 2nd ed. New York: Oxford University Press, 1973; Ashley Montagu, *The Na-ture of Human Aggression*. New York: Oxford University Press, 1976; Ashley Montagu, *Learning Non-Aggression.* New York: Oxford University Press, 1978. Robert A. Hinde, *Biological Bases of Human Social Behaviour.* New York: McGraw-Hill, 1974: Richard E. Leakey and Roger Lewin, *Origins*. New York: E. P. Dutton, 1977; Joan Marble Cook, *In Defense of Homo Sapiens*. New York: Farrar, Straus & Giroux, 1975; Robert Claiborne, *God or Beast: Evolution and Human Nature,* New York: W. W. Norton, 1974.

:26–29   J. B. S. Haldane, *The Causes of Evolution*. 2nd ed. London: Longmans, 1932, p. 131.

:29–32   J. Z. Young, op. cit., 1971, p. 480.

88:11–13   John Nance, *The Gentle Tasaday*. New York: Harcourt Brace Jovanovich, 1975.

:23–25   Alice Brues, "The Spearman and the Archer—An Essay on Selection in Body Build," *American Anthropologist,* vol. 61, 1960, pp. 457–469.

:26–35   J. H. Crook, "Sexual Selection, Dimorphism, and Social Orga-nization in the Primates," in *Sexual Selection and the Des-cent of Man, 1871–1971*. Chicago: Aldine Publishing Co., 1972, p. 271 and p. 273.

88:39 to   C. H. Waddington, *The Ethical Animal*. New York: Atheneum,
89:1–3   1961.

:4–11   Ashley Montagu, *On Being Human*. 2nd ed. New York: Haw-thorn Books, 1966.

Page and line

:11–19   J. Z. Young, *The Life of Vertebrates.* 2nd ed. Oxford: the Clarendon Press, 1962, pp. 640–641.

:20–34   J. Z. Young, ibid., p. 651.

89:39 to   Adolph Portmann, *Biologische Fragmente.* Basel: Benno
90:1   Schwalbe & Co., 1944.

:1–2   John Bostock, "Exterior Gestation, Primitive Sleep, Enuresis and Asthma: Study in Aetiology," *Medical Journal of Australia,* vol. 2, 1958, pp. 149–153, pp. 185–188.

:2–3   F. Kovács, "Biological Interpretation of the Nine-Month Duration of Human Pregnancy," *Acta Biologica Magyar, Tudom. Akad.,* vol. 10, 1960, pp. 331–336.

:3   Ashley Montagu, "The Origin and Significance of Neonatal and Infant Immaturity," *Journal of the American Medical Association,* vol. 178, 1961, pp. 156–157.

:9–11   Stephen Jay Gould, *Ontogeny and Phylogeny.* Cambridge: Harvard University Press, 1977, p. 369.

:11–12   R. E. Passingham, "Changes in the Size and Organization of the Brain in Man and His Ancestors," *Brain, Behavior and Evolution,* vol. 11, 1975, pp. 73–90.

:15–18   Adolph Portmann, op. cit.

:18–24   F. Kovács, op. cit.

:24–39   John Bostock, op. cit.

91:16–19   John Bostock, op. cit., p. 12.

:28–31   John Bostock, op. cit., p. 13.

92:30 to   Ashley Montagu, *On Being Human.* 2nd ed. New York: Haw-
93:1–9   thorn Books, 1966.

:9–12   Weston LaBarre, *The Ghost Dance.* New York: Doubleday, 1970.

:25–40   Ashley Montagu, *The Direction of Human Development.* 2nd ed. New York: Hawthorn Books, 1970.

:13–19   Robert Gray Patton and Lytt I. Gardner, *Growth Failure in Maternal Deprivation.* Springfield, Illinois: C C Thomas, 1963; John Bowlby, *Maternal Care and Mental Health.* Geneva World Health Organization, 1951; various authors, *Deprivation of Maternal Care: A Reassessment of Its Effects.* Geneva: World Health Organization, 1962; John Bowlby, *Attachment and Loss,* 3 volumes. New York: Basic Books, 1969/1973/1980.

:21–22   Charles Sanders Peirce, "Evolutionary Love," *The Monist,* vol. 3, 1893, pp. 176–200; reprinted in the collection of Peirce's essays, *Chance, Love, & Logic.* New York: Braziller, 1956, pp. 267–300.

:22   Petr Kropotkin, *Mutual Aid.* London: 1902; Boston: Porter Sargent, 1955.

:23–25   Robert Ardrey, *African Genesis.* New York: Athenum, 1961;

Page and line

Konrad Lorenz, *On Aggression.* New York: Harcourt, Brace & World, 1963.

:23–25   Ashley Montagu, *Darwin, Competition, and Cooperation.* New York: Henry Schuman, 1952, Reprinted, Westport, Conn.: Greenwood Press, 1973; Richard E. Leakey and Roger Lewin, *People of the Lake: Mankind and Its Beginnings.* New York: Anchor Press/Doubleday, 1978; Richard B. Lee and Irven De Vore, *Man the Hunter.* Chicago: Aldine Publishing Co., 1968; Carleton S. Coon, *The Hunting Peoples.* Boston: Little, Brown, 1971; Elman R. Service, *The Hunters.* Englewood Cliffs, New Jersey: Prentice-Hall, 1966.

93:30–35   Hermann J. Muller, "Genetics in the Scheme of Things," *Proceedings of the Eighth International Congress of Genetics (Hereditas Supplementary Volume),* 1949, pp. 96–125. Ashley Montagu, "Of Man, Animals, and Morals," *Journal of the National Association for the Advancement of Humane Education,* vol. 1, 1974, pp. 1–8. Ashley Montagu, "Wilderness and Humanity," in *Wilderness in a Changing World,* Bruce M. Kilgore (ed.), San Francisco: Sierra Club, 1966, pp. 220–227; Ashley Montagu, "Is Man Innately Aggressive? in *On the Fifth Day: Animal Rights and Human Ethics,* Richard Knowles Morris and Michael W. Fox (eds.), Washington: Acropolis Books, 1978, pp. 93–110: Henry G. Maurice, *Ask Now the Beasts.* London: Society for the Preservation of the Fauna of the Empire, 1948; Stanley and Rosalind Godlovitch and John Harris (eds.), *Animals, Men and Morals.* New York: Taplinger Co., 1972.

93:36–40   Ashley Montagu (ed.), *The Practice of Love.* Englewood Cliffs: Prentice-Hall, 1975; Ashley Montagu, (ed.), *Culture and Human Development.* Englewood Cliffs: Prentice-Hall, 1974; Ian D. Suttie, *The Origins of Love and Hate.* New York: Agora Softback, 1966; Ashley Montagu, *The Direction of Human Development.* 2nd ed. New York: Hawthorn Books, 1970; M. Bevan-Brown, *The Sources of Love and Fear.* New York: Vanguard Press, 1950.

94:13–33   Ashley Montagu, "Mother's Touch," *Science Digest,* vol. 89, 1981, p. 16.

95:18–40   Otto Rank, *The Trauma of Birth.* New York: Robert Brunner, 1952. Originally published in German in 1924, and in English translation in 1929.

98:16–19   Ashley Montagu and Floyd Matson, *The Human Connection.* New York: McGraw-Hill, 1979.

:19–40   W. S. Condon and W. D. Ogston, "Sound Film Analysis of Normal and Pathological Behavior Patterns," *Journal of Nervous and Mental Diseases,* vol. 143, 1966, pp. 338–347.

:31–40   W. S. Condon and L. W. Sander, "Neonate Movement Is Syn-

Page and line

chronized with Adult Speech: Interactional Participation and Language Acquisition," *Science,* vol. 183, 1974, pp. 99–101.

99:2–3   A. A. Tomatis, *Éducation et Dyslexie.* Paris: Les Éditions ESF, 1972.

99:2–3   H. M. Truby, "Prenatal and Neonatal Speech, 'Pre-Speech,' and an Infantile-Speech Lexicon," *Word,* vol. 27, 1971, pp. 57–101.

:4–32   Lee Salk, "The Effects of the Normal Heartbeat Sound on the Behavior of the Newborn Infant: Implications for Mental Health," *World Mental Health,* vol. 12, 1960, pp. 1–8, also "Sound of Love," *American Weekly,* 21 Aug 1960, p. 4.

100:12–28   Kaye Lowman, "A Legacy of Love," *La Leche League News* (Jubilee Year 1956–1981), vol. 23, no. 1, 1981, pp. 1–24.

101:14–21   Harry F. Harlow, *Learning to Love.* New York: Ballantine Books, 1971; Thelma Rowell, *Social Behavior of Monkeys.* Baltimore: Penguin Books, 1972; Harriet L. Rheingold (ed.), *Maternal Behavior in Mammals.* New York: John Wiley & Sons, 1963; Jane Van Lawick-Goodall, *In the Shadow of Man.* Boston: Houghton Mifflin Co., 1971.

101:37 to   Lorna Marshall, *The !Kung of Nyae Nyae.* Cambridge: Harvard
102:1–4   University Press, 1976.

:8–16   Ibid., pp. 316–318.

104:18–23   J. P. Greenhill, *Obstetrics.* 13th ed. Philadelphia: W. B. Saunders, 1965, pp. 376–377.

105:3–12   K. Robson, "The Role of Eye-to-Eye Contact in Maternal-Infant Attachment," *Journal of Child Psychiatry,* vol. 8, 1967, pp. 13–25.

:31–37   Betsy Marvin McKinney, "The Effects upon the Mother of Removal of the Infant Immediately after Birth," *Child-Family Digest,* vol. 10, 1954, pp. 63–65.

106:34–37   Glenn Collins, "Friendship: A Fact of Life for Toddlers Too," *The New York Times,* Monday, 15 December 1980, p. B16; Zick Rubin, *Children's Friendships,* Cambridge: Harvard University Press, 1980; Robert Selman and Jeanne Brooks-Gunn, *Social Cognition and the Acquisition of Self,* New York: Plenum Press, 1980.

107:7–17   *Ritualization,* a term coined by Julian Huxley to describe the courtship display of the great crested grebe. J. S. Huxley, "Courtship Activities in the Red-Throated Diver (*Colymbus stellatus*): Together with a Discussion of the Evolution of Courtship in Birds," *Journal of the Linnaean Society of London, Zoology,* vol. 53, 1923, pp. 253–192.

107:24–33   Irenäus Eibl-Eibesfeldt, *Love and Hate: The Natural History of*

Page and line

              Behavior Patterns. New York: Holt, Rinehart & Winston, 1972, p. 152.

108:2–14   Mary Midgley, *Beast and Man: The Roots of Human Nature*. Ithaca, N.Y.: Cornell University Press, p. 333.

109:6–23   Alfred Adler, *Social Interest: A Challenge to Mankind*. New York: 1938, p. 214, pp. 220–221.

109:24–30   M. Bevan Brown, *The Sources of Love and Fear*. New York: Vanguard Press, 1950, p. 15.

110:37 to   Lisa F. Berkman, "Social Ties and Length of Life," *Science*
111:1–8   *News*, vol. 118, 1980, p. 392.

112:19–23   Emory S. Bogardus, Discussion, in "The Groups Fallacy in Relation to Social Science," Floyd H. Allport (ed.), *American Journal of Sociology*, vol. 29, 1924, p. 704.

:23–27   Harry S. Sullivan, "The Illusion of Personal Individuality," *Psychiatry*, vol. 13, 1950, p. 329.

:28–30   Alfred North Whitehead, *Adventures in Ideas*. New York: Cambridge University Press, 1933, p. 137.

:30–34   E. Gutkind, *Choose Life*. New York: Henry Schuman, 1952, p. 134.

:30 to   C. M. Child, "The Beginnings of Unity and Order in Living
113:1–4   Things," in E. Dummer (ed.), *The Unconscious*. New York: Alfred A. Knopf, 1927, p. 37.

:27–35   V. J. Bourke, "Will in Western Thought." In William K. Frankena, *Ethics*. 2nd ed. Englewood Cliffs, New Jersey: Prentice-Hall, 1973.

115:4–6   F. R. Tennant, *The Sources of the Doctrines of the Fall and Original Sin*. New York: Schocken Books, 1968; Eric Smith, *Some Versions of the Fall*. Pittsburgh: University of Pittsburgh Press, 1973.

4. THE CHILD

116:11–21   Louis MacNeice, "Prayer before Birth," In *Eighty-Five Poems*. London: Faber & Faber, 1959, pp. 121–122.

118:25 to   Edward Glover, *The Roots of Crime*. New York: Schocken
119:1–7   Books, 1970, p. 8.

:11–19   Ashley Montagu, *The Direction of Human Development*. 2nd ed. New York: Hawthorn Books, 1970.

:33 to   E. Richard Sorenson, *The Edge of the Forest*. Washington,
120:1–17   D.C.: Smithsonian Institution Press, 1976.

:19–21   Ashley Montagu (ed.), *Learning Non-Aggression*. New York: Oxford University Press, 1978.

:32 to   Herbert J. Muller, *The Uses of the Past*. New York: Oxford
121:1–3   University Press, 1952, p. 160.

122:27–23   Edith Cobb, *The Ecology of Imagination in Childhood*. New York: Columbia University Press, 1977, p. 95.

Page and line

123:7–13   Ashley Montagu (ed.), *Culture and Human Development*. En-
            glewood Cliffs, New Jersey: Prentice-Hall, 1974.

:35 to   William A. Mason, "Early Social Deprivation in the Nonhuman
124:1–5   Primates: Implications for Human Behavior," in David C.
            Glass (ed.) *Environmental Influences*. New York: Rocke-
            feller University Press, 1968, pp. 70–101.

124:13 to   Ashley Montagu, *The Reproductive Development of the Fe-
125:1–16   male*. 2nd ed. Littleton, Mass.: PSG Publishing Co., 1979.

:3–11   B. T. Donovan and J. J. Van der Werff ten Bosch, *Physiology of
            Puberty*. London: Edward Arnold, 1965: M. M. Grumbach
            et al. (eds.), *Control of Onset of Puberty*. New York: John
            Wiley & Sons, 1974; H. E. Kulin, "Physiology of Adoles-
            cence in Man," *Human Biology*, vol. 46, 1974, pp. 133–144.

126:39 to   David Brewster, *Memoirs of the Life, Writings and Discoveries
127:1–3   of Sir Isaac Newton*, 2 volumes. New York: Johnston Re-
            print Corp., 1965, p. 407.

:30–31   Ashley Montagu and Floyd Matson, *The Human Connection*.
            New York: McGraw-Hill, 1979.

128:3–13   John Fiske, "The Meaning of Infancy," in *Excursions of an
            Evolutionist*. Boston: Houghton, Mifflin & Co., 1892, p.
            319.

5. THE NEOTENOUS TRAITS OF THE CHILD

132:11–12   *The New English Bible*. New York & London: Oxford Univer-
            sity Press and Cambridge University Press, 1970. *The New
            Testament*, p. 221. This is a more faithful translation than
            the Authorized Version in the language of the present.

:26–33   Edith Cobb, *The Ecology of Imagination in Childhood*. New
            York: Columbia University Press, 1977, p. 59.

134:15–22   Zick Rubin, *Children's Friendships*. Cambridge: Harvard Uni-
            versity Press, 1980.

:27–38   Robert L. Selman and Jeanne Brooks-Gunn, *Social Cognition
            and the Acquisition of Self*. New York: Plenum Press, 1980;
            Robert L. Selman and Anne P. Selman, "Children's Ideas
            about Friendship: A New Theory." *Psychology Today*, Oc-
            tober 1979, pp. 71–80, 114; Robert L. Selman, "The Child
            as a Friendship Philosopher," in *The Development of
            Friendship*. Cambridge: Harvard University Press, 1981;
            Robert L. Selman, *The Growth of Interpersonal Under-
            standing: Developmental and Clinical Studies*. New York:
            Academic Press, 1980.

:39 to   Robert L. Selman and Jeanne Brooks-Gunn, op. cit.
135:1–2

Page and line

:6–8   Robert L. Selman, quoted in Glenn Collins, "Friendship: A
                Fact of Life for Toddlers, Too." *The New York Times,* 15
                December 1980, p. B16.

137:11–17   David Bakan, *Sigmund Freud and the Jewish Mystical Tradition.*
                Princeton, N.J.: D. Van Nostrand Co., 1958.

:28–36   G. Carpenter, "Mother's Face and the Newborn," in *Child
                Alive,* R. Lewin (ed.), New York: Doubleday, 1975;
                T. G. R. Bower, *The Perceptual World of the Child.* Cam-
                bridge: Harvard University Press, 1977.

145:34–35   D. K. Spelt, "The Conditioning of the Human Fetus in Utero,"
                Journal of Experimental Psychology, vol. 38, 1948, pp.
                338–346.

149:1–8   John Stuart Mill, *Autobiography.* London: Longmans, 1873, p.
                142.

152:24–28   Plutarch, *Moralia* III, p. 315.

:33–39   Thomas Hobbes, *Leviathan.* London: Andrew Crooke, 1651.
                For the best modern edition see Thomas Hobbes,
                Leviathan, edited with an introduction by Michael
                Oakeshott, Oxford: Basil Blackwell, 1955.

:20–32   Edith Cobb, op. cit., p. 27.

154:11–23   Erik H. Erikson, *Toys and Reasons: Stages in the Ritualization
                of Experience.* New York: W. W. Norton, 1977, p. 17.

155:36–37   Alfred B. Garrett, *The Flash of Genius.* Princeton, N.J.: D.
                Van Nostrand Co., 1963.

156:13–14   W. H. Thorpe, *Animal Nature and Human Nature.* New York:
                Anchor Press/Doubleday, 1974.

:35–39   Hans Vaihinger, *The Philosophy of "As If."* London: Kegan
                Paul, 1924.

157:8–16   Roger Fry, *Vision and Design.* London: Chatto & Windus,
                1920/28, p. 96.

:12–16   Roger Fry, op. cit., p. 20.

159:10–20   Jerome Singer, *The Child's World of Make-Believe.* New York:
                Academic Press, 1973, pp. 258–259.

160:20–23   J. W. Getzels and P. W. Jackson, *Creativity and Intelligence:
                Explorations with Gifted Students.* New York: John Wiley &
                Sons., 1962; J. P. Guilford, *The Nature of Human Intelli-
                gence.* New York: McGraw-Hill, 1967; Michael A. Wal-
                lach, "Creativity," in Paul H. Mussen (ed.), *Carmichael's
                Manual of Child Psychology.* 3rd ed., New York: John
                Wiley & Sons, 1970, vol. 1, pp. 1211–1272; Michael Wal-
                lach, *The Intelligence/Creativity Distinction.* New York:
                General Learning Press, 1971.

160:24 to   J. P. Guilford, *The Nature of Human Intelligence.* New York:
162:1–2   McGraw-Hill, 1967.

:26–35   L. E. Abt and Stanley Rosner (eds.), *The Creative Experience.*
                New York: Grossman, 1970.

Page and line

163:37 to   Jerome Singer, op. cit., pp. 72, 154.
164:1–7

:8–24   R. Helson, "Childhood Interest Clusters Related to Creativity
                 in Women," *Journal of Consulting Psychology,* vol. 29,
                 1965, pp. 253–361; R. Helson, "Personality Characteristics
                 and Developmental History of Creative College Women,"
                 Genetic Psychology Monographs, vol. 76, 1967, pp. 205–
                 266; Jerome Singer, op. cit., pp. 254–255, 228.

:25–27   Jerome Singer, op. cit., p. 246.

:34–39   René Dubos, *Man Adapting.* New Haven: Yale University
                 Press, 1965, p. xviii.

165:7–9   William Wordsworth, *The Prelude.* 1850.

:23–28   Jerome Singer, op. cit., p. 259.

166:30 to   For excellent summaries of Piaget's many-volumed work see
167:1–36   his own Jean Piaget and Bärbel Inhelder, *The Psychology
                 of the Child.* New York: Basic Books, 1969, and perhaps
                 the even more thorough work by Dorothy E. Singer and
                 Tracey A. Revenson, *A Piaget Primer: How a Child
                 Thinks.* New York: International Universities Press, 1978.

167:36 to   Antoine de St. Exupéry, *The Little Prince.* New York: Reynal,
168:1–9   1943.

:27–35   Matthew Arnold, "A Speech at Eton," in *Irish Essays.* London:
                 Smith Elder & Co., 1882.

171:14–20   Reuven Kohen-Raz, *Psychobiological Aspects of Cognitive
                 Growth.* New York: Academic Press, 1977, pp. 46–47.

173:38 to   Ashley Montagu (ed.), *Culture and Human Development.* En-
174:1–11   glewood Cliffs, N.J.: Prentice-Hall, 1974; Ashley Montagu,
                 The Direction of Human Development. 2nd ed., New York:
                 Hawthorn Books, 1970; A. M. Clarke and A. D. B. Clarke,
                 Early Experience. Myth and Evidence. New York: Free
                 Press, 1976.

175:15–16   Jeffrey H. Goldstein and Paul E. McGhee (eds.), *The Psychol-
                 ogy of Humor.* New York: Academic Press, 1972.

176:16–31   William Wordsworth, *The Prelude,* 1805/06. There is a much
                 revised version of this posthumously published in 1850.

178:32 to   Yvonne Brackbill, "Extinction of Smiling Response in Infants
179:1–5   as a Function of Reinforcement Schedule," *Child Devel-
                 opment,* vol. 29, 1958, pp. 114–124; J. L. Gewirtz, "The
                 Course of Infant Smiling in Four Child-Rearing Environ-
                 ments," in *Determinants of Infant Behaviour III.* B. M.
                 Foss (ed.). New York: John Wiley & Sons, 1968; William
                 C. Sheppard and Robert H. Willoughby, *Child Behavior:
                 Learning and Development.* New York: Rand McNally,
                 1975, pp. 263–272.

180:1–16   E. Richard Sorenson, *The Edge of the Forest.* Washington,
                 D.C.: Smithsonian Institution Press, 1977; E. Richard

Page and line

Sorenson, "Cooperation and Freedom among the Fore of New Guinea, in *Learning Non-Aggression,* Ashley Montagu (ed.), New York: Oxford University Press, 1978, pp. 12–30.

:17–21   A. R. Radcliffe-Brown, *The Andaman Islanders.* Cambridge: At the University Press, 1922/1933, p. 241.

:22–28   Ashley Montagu, *The Human Revolution.* New York: Bantam Books, 1967. Saree Penbharkkul and Samuel Karelitz, "Lacrimation in the Neonatal and Early Infancy Period of Premature and Full-Term Infants," *Journal of Pediatrics,* vol. 61, 1962, pp. 859–863; Leonard Apt and Bruce F. Cullen, "Newborns Do Secrete Tears," *Journal of the American Medical Association,* vol. 9, 1964, pp. 951–953.

181:13–16 Ashley Montagu, *Touching: The Human Significance of the Skin.* 2nd ed., New York: Harper & Row, 1978, pp. 205 sq.

:23–32   Lionel Tiger, *Optimism.* New York: Simon & Schuster, 1979.

181:38 to Fred C. Kelly, *The Wright Brothers.* New York: Harcourt,
182:1–11   Brace & Co., 1943. Harry Combs, *Kill Devil Hill: Discovering the Secret of the Wright Brothers.* Boston: Houghton Mifflin Co., 1979.

185:4–12   Julia Gordon, *My Country School Diary.* New York: Dell, 1971.

:14–15   Edward Westermarck, *The Origin and Development of Moral Ideas.* vol. 2, pp. 117 sq. London: Macmillan, 1917.

:15–19   Francis Hutcheson, *System of Moral Philosophy.* 2 vols., London, 1755, vol. 2, p. 28.

:20–25   G. Stanley Hall, "Children's Lies," *American Journal of Psychology,* vol. 3, 1890/91, pp. 59–70.

186:31–40 Edith Cobb, *The Ecology of Imagination in Childhood.* New York: Columbia University Press, 1977. p. 111.

187:5–18   Robert Browning, *Paracelsus.* London: Effingham Wilson, 1835.

:20 to   Ashley Montagu, *The Nature of Human Aggression.* New York:
188:1–23   Oxford University Press, 1976.

:36 to   W. S. Condon and L. A. Sander, "Neonate Movement Is Syn-
189:1–6   chronized with Adult Speech: Interactional Participation and Language Acquisition," *Science,* vol. 183, 1974, pp. 99–101. See also M. Bullowa, "When Infant and Adult Communicate, How Do They Synchronize Their Behaviors?" In Adam Kendon et al. (eds.), *Organization of Behavior in Face-to-Face Interaction.* Chicago: Aldine, 1975, pp. 96–129.

189:26–29 Judith L. Hanna, *To Dance Is Human.* Austin: University of Texas Press, 1979, p. 19.

:34 to   John M. Chernoff, "Music-Making Children of Africa,"
190:1–17   *Natural History,* vol. 88, 1979, pp. 68–75; John M. Cher-

Page and line

noff, *African Rhythm and African Sensibility*. Chicago: University of Chicago Press, 1979.

:29–31   Plato, *Laws*. Book 7:803 D–E.

:31–39   Plato, ibid., Book 7, 795E.

191:36–39   Havelock Ellis, *The Dance of Life*. London: Constable, 1923.

192:1–9   Cyril W. Beaumont, *The Diaghilev Ballet in London: A Personal Record*. 3rd ed. London: Adam & Charles Black, 1951.

:9–12   Richard Buckle, *Diaghilev*. New York: Atheneum, 1979; Arnold L. Haskell, *Diaghileff: His Artistic and Private Life*. London: Gollancz, 1947; Arnold L. Haskell, *Ballet*. London: Penguin Books, 1938.

:23–24   Alice Kehoe, "Ritual and Religions," Paper prepared for the IXth International Congress of Anthropology and International Sciences, Chicago, 1973, p. 7.

:28–29   Plato, *Laws*. Book 7, 795E.

193:28–34   Richard Edwardes, *A Song of the Lute*. 1563. Shakespeare used a version of this song in *Romeo and Juliet*.

6. THOSE WHOM THE GODS LOVE

194:2–3   A play upon the oft-quoted line "Those whom the gods love die young," one of the three surviving lines from the play *The Double Deceiver* by Menander (343 B.C.–329 B.C.), the Attic playwright.

198:26–38   John Stuart Mill, *On Liberty*. London: John W. Parker, 1859.

202:17 to   Gay Gaer Luce, *Your Second Life*. New York: Delacorte
203:1–18   Press/Seymour Lawrence, 1979.

:13–14   Gay Gaer Luce, ibid., p. 17.

Jaap Goudsmit et al., "Evidence For and Against the Transmissibility of Alzheimer Disease," *Neurology*, vol. 30, 1980, pp. 945–950; N. B. Rewcastle, C. J. Gibbs, Jr., and D. C. Gajdusek, "Transmission of Familial Alzheimer's Disease to Primates," *Journal of Neuropathology and Experimental Neurology*, vol. 37, 1978, p. 679; Peter Davies/Harold M. Schmeck, Jr., "Research Attempts to Fight Senility," *The New York Times*, 21 July 1979, p. C1.

204:23–28   Bernard L. Strehler, "A New Age for Aging," *Natural History*, February 1973, pp. 18, 82–85.

:29–34   National Institute on Aging, *Recent Developments in Clinical and Research Geriatric Medicine: The NIA Role*. Bethesda, Md: National Institutes of Health, Publication No. 80-1990, 1980.

205:2–23   Bernard L. Strehler, ibid., pp. 84–85.

206:14–16   Frances Tenenbaum, *Over 55 Is Not Illegal*. Boston: Houghton Mifflin Co., 1979, p. 5; Morton A. Leberman, *Time*, 21 November 1973.

Page and line

207:14–29   Robert Butler, *Why Survive? Growing Old in America.* New York: Harper & Row, 1973.

209:17–29   J. E. Birren, *Aging: Prospects and Issues.* Los Angeles: University of Southern California Press, 1973.

:36 to   G. G. Haydu, "Aging and Experience Forms," *New York State*
210:1–2   *Journal of Medicine,* vol. 75, 1975, p. 1556.

:3–8   Lawrence Galton, *The Truth about Senility.* New York: Thomas Y. Crowell, 1939; Alexander Leaf, *Youth in Old Age.* New York: McGraw-Hill, 1975.

:16–22   Marian C. Diamond, "The Aging Brain: Some Enlightening and Optimistic Results," *American Scientist,* vol. 66, 1978, pp. 66–71.

:22–25   W. M. Cowan, "Neuronal Death as a Regulative Mechanism in the Control of Cell Number in the Nervous System," *Development and Aging in the Nervous System,* M. Rockstein (ed.), New York: Academic Press, 1973, pp. 19–37.

211:10 to   David Hackett Fischer, *Growing Old in America.* New York:
212:1–10   Oxford University Press, 1977, pp. 204–205.

:20–34   Harold Brody, "Organization of the Cerebral Cortex," *Journal of Comparative Neurology,* vol. 102, 1955, pp. 517–557.

214:28 to   David A. Levitsky (ed.), *Malnutrition, Environment and Behav-*
215:1–4   *ior.* Ithaca, N.Y.: Cornell University Press, 1979. Also see Ashley Montagu's review, "Not By Bread Alone," in *The Sciences,* September 1979, pp. 23–24.

214:to   Ashley Montagu, "Sociogenic Brain Damage," *American An-*
215:1–4   *thropologist,* vol. 74, 1972, pp. 1045–1061.

:5–23   Florida Scott-Maxwell, "We Are the Sum of Our Days," *The Listener* (London), 14 October 1954, pp. 627–628.

:25–39   Ronald Blythe, *The View in Winter.* New York: Harcourt Brace Jovanovich. 1979.

216:24–26   David Hackett Fischer, op. cit.; Margaret Hellie Huyck, *Growing Older.* Englewood Cliffs, New Jersey: Prentice-Hall, 1974.

217:16–18   Ashley Montagu, *The Direction of Human Development.* 2nd ed. New York: Hawthorn Books 1970; Ashley Montagu, *On Being Human.* 2nd ed. New York: Hawthorn Books. 1966: Ashley Montagu and Floyd Matson, *The Human Connection.* New York, 1979.

:24–28   Dan Georgakas, *The Methuselah Factors: Living Long and Living Well.* New York: Simon & Schuster, 1981.

7. IMPORT

219:23–26   Simone de Beauvoir, *Old Age.* London: Andre Deutsch, 1972.

220:20–33   W. D. Hambly, *Origins of Education among Primitive Peoples.* London: Macmillan, 1926; Nathan Miller, *The Child in*

Primitive Society. New York: Brentano's, 1928; Murray L. Wax et al. (eds.), *Anthropological Perspectives on Education.* New York: Basic Books, 1971.

222:23–26 Walter de la Mare, *Early One Morning: Chapters on Children and Childhood as It Is Revealed in Particular in Early Memories and in Early Writings.* London: Faber & Faber, 1935.

223:29–30 Richard C. Adelman, "Definition of Biological Aging," in *Epidemiology of Aging,* Suzanne G. Haynes and Manning Feinleib (eds.), Bethesda, Md.: National Institute on Aging, 1980, pp. 9–13.

224:10–12 J. E. Blum and L. F. Jarvick, "Intellectual Performance of Octogenarians as a Function of Education and Initial Ability," *Human Development,* vol. 17, 1975, p. 364.

224:18–23 T. J. Carlo, "Recreation Participation Patterns and Successful Aging," *Journal of Gerontology,* vol. 29, p. 416; Peter P. Lamy, *Prescribing for the Elderly.* Littleton, Mass.: PSG Publishing Co., 1980, pp. 41–43.

APPENDIX A: A HISTORY OF NEOTENY

225:1–12 Julius Kollmann, "Das Ueberwintern von europäischen Frosch- und Tritonlarven und die Umwandlung des mexikanischen axolotl," *Verhandlungen der naturforschenden Gesellschaft,* Basel, vol. 7, 1884, pp. 384–394.

:12–15 Auguste Duméril "Métamorphoses des Batraciens Urodèles à Branchies Extérieurs du Mexique dits Axolotls, Observées à la Menagérie des Reptiles du Muséum d'Histoire Naturelle," Annales des Sciences Naturelles Zoölogiques," vol. 7, 1867, pp. 229–254.

226:19:30 Karl E. von Baer, "Über Prof. Nic. Wagner's Entdeckung von Larven, die Sich Fortpflanzen, Herren Garren's Verwandte und Ergänzende Beobachtung und Über die Pädogenesis überhaupt," *Bulletin d'Académie Imperiale des Sciences St. Petersbourg,* vol. 9, 1866, pp. 63–137.

:36 to
227:1–10 Hans Gadow, *Amphibia and Reptiles.* London: Macmillan, 1901, p. 65.

:14 to
229:1–12 Edwin Drinker Cope, "On the Origin of Genera," *Proceedings of the Philadelphia Academy of Natural Sciences,* vol. 20, 1868, pp. 242–300, and published separately by the author in 1869. Reprinted in E. D. Cope, *The Origin of the Fittest.* New York: Appleton, 1887, p. 43.

227:18 to
228:1–14 Charles Darwin, *The Origin of Species.* 6th ed. London: 1872, p. 160.

:1–14 Edwin Drinker Cope, *The Origin of the Fittest,* p. 11.

Page and line

:1–12   Edwin Drinker Cope, "The Hypothesis of Evolution: Physical and Metaphysical," *Lippincott's Magazine,* vol. 6, 1870, pp. 173–180. Reprinted in Cope, 1887, pp. 146–147, p. 154.

:16 to   Edwin Drinker Cope, op. cit., 1887, pp. 161–162.

229:1–5   Phyllis Grosskurth, *Havelock Ellis: A Biography.* New York:
:21   Alfred A. Knopf, 1980.

:21–24   Havelock Ellis, *Studies in the Psychology of Sex.* Philadelphia. F. A. Davis, 7 volumes, 1901–1928 (*Sexual Inversion.* Watford: University Press, 1897).

:29–30   Havelock Ellis, *Man and Woman: A Study of Human Secondary Characters.* London: Walter Scott, 1894, p. 26.

:36–39   Ibid., p. 26.

230:1–4   Ibid., pp. 27–28.

:5–9   Ibid., p. 26.

      Ibid., p. 518 and 519.

231:1–6   Boas, J. E. V., "Über Neotenie," *Festschrift Für Carl Gegenbaur.* Leipzig: W. Engelmann, vol. 2, pp. 1–20.

:7–9   O. Jaekel, "Über Verschiedene Wege Phylogenetischer Entwicklung," *Verhandlungen des V. Internationalen Zoologen-Congresses.* Berlin, 1901.

:10–12   Alfred Giard, "La Poecilogenie," *Bulletin Biologique de la France et de la Belgique,* vol. 39, 1905, pp. 15301–187.

:12–15   J. H. F. Kohlbrugge, *Die Morphologische Abstammung der Menschen.* Stuttgart, 1908.

:16–24   Adam Sedgwick, "The Influence of Darwin on the Study of Animal Embryology," In *Darwin and Modern Science,* A. C. Seward (ed.), Cambridge: at the University Press, 1909, pp. 178–179. See also, Adam Sedgwick, "On the Law of Development Commonly Known as von Baer's Law, and on the Significance of Ancestral Rudiments in Embryonic Development," *Quarterly Journal of Microscopical Science,* vol. 36, 1894, pp. 35–52.

:31–36   Adam Sedgwick, op. cit., 1909, p. 182.

232:16–33 Ernst Haeckel, *Anthropogenie.* Berlin: Georg Reimer, 1874.

:24 to   Walter Garstang, "The Theory of Recapitulation: A Critical
233:1–3   Restatement of the Biogenetic Law," *Journal of the Linnaean Society, Zoology,* vol. 35, 1922, pp. 81–101.

:7–13   Theodosius Dobzhansky, Review of *Evolution as a Process.* J. S. Huxley, A. C. Hardy, and E. B. Ford (eds.), London: Allen & Unwin, 1954; in *Science,* vol. 121, 1955, pp. 162–163.

:24–29   Arthur Keith, "The Adaptational Machinery Concerned in the Evolution of Man's Body," *Nature,* 18 August 1923, Sup-
:29–31   plement. Arthur Keith, "Capital as a Factor in Evolution," *Rationalist Annual,* 1925, p. 10; Arthur Keith, "The Differentiation of Mankind into Racial Types, *Report of the British*

Page and line

	Assoc. Adv. Sci. London: John Murray, 1919/1920, pp. 275–281.
:34 to 233:1–5	Alister C. Hardy, "Escape from Specialization," in *Evolution as Process.* J. S. Huxley, A. C. Hardy, and E. B. Ford (eds.). London: Allen & Unwin, 1945, p. 139.
234:10 to 239:1–39	Louis Bolk, *Die Morphogenie der Primatenzähne. Eine Weitere Begründung und Ausarbeitung der Dimer-Theorie.* Jena: Gustav Fischer, 1914.
234:20 to 235:1–8	Louis Bolk, "On the Character of Morphological Modifications in Consequence of Affections of the Endocrine Organs," *Proceedings of the Koninklijke Nederlandse Akademie van Wetenschappen,* vol. 23, 1922, pp. 1328–1338.
:8–17	Louis Bolk, "The Part Played by the Endocrine Glands in the Evolution of Man," *The Lancet,* 10 September 1921.
:12–17	Louis Bolk, "On the Significance of the Supraorbital Ridges in the Primates," *Proc. Kon. Akad. Wetensch. Amsterdam,* vol. 25, 1923, pp. 16–20.
234:36 to 235:1–6	Louis Bolk, "On the Character of Morphological Modifications . . . ," op. cit., 1922, pp. 1329–1330.
:16–17	Louis Bolk, "On the Significance of the Supraorbital Ridges . . . , op. cit., 1923, p. 21.
:18–21	Louis Bolk, "The Problem of Orthognathism," *Proc. Kon. Akad. Wetensch. Amsterdam,* vol. 25, 1923, pp. 371–380.
:21–23	Louis Bolk, "The Chin Problem," *Proc. Kon. Akad. Wetensch. Amsterdam,* vol. 27, 1924, pp. 329–324.
:24–33	Louis Bolk, "The Problem of Anthropogenesis," *Proc. Kon. Akad. Wetensch. Amsterdam,* vol. 29, 1926, pp. 465–475.
:28–33	Louis Bolk, ibid., p. 9; "The Problem of Anthropogenesis," p. 469.
:28–33	Louis Bolk, *Das Problem der Menschwerdung,* p. 8; "The Problem of Anthropogenesis," p. 469.
:34sq.	Louis Bolk, *Das Problem der Menschwerdung.* Jena: Gustav Fischer, 1926.
239:22–24	Marcellin Boule and Henri Vallois, *Fossil Men: A Textbook of Human Palaeontology.*
:11–14	For a thorough critical demolition of Bolk's hormone theory of evolution, see Solly Zuckerman, "Hormones and Evolution," *Man,* vol. 36, 1936, pp. 129–135.
:30–33	Ashley Montagu, *The Reproductive Development of the Female.* 3rd ed. Littleton, Mass.: PSG Publishing Co., 1979.
240:1–10	M. R. Drennan, *A Short Course on Physical Anthropology.* Cape Town: Mercantile Press, 1937, p. 59.
:6–10	M. R. Drennan, "Note on the Morphological Status of the Swanscombe and Fontèchevade Skulls," *American Journal of Physical Anthropology,* vol. 14, 1956, pp. 73–84.

Page and line

:15–19   O. H. Schindewolf, "Das Problem der Menschwerdung, ein Paläontologischer Lösungsversuch," *Jb. Preuss. Geol. Landesanst.* vol. 49, 1929, pp. 716–766.

:18–19   O. H. Schindewolf, *Paläontologie, Entwicklungslehre und Genetik: Kritik und Synthese.* Berlin: Bonträger, 1936.

:28 to   Gavin de Beer, *Embryology and Evolution.* Oxford: the Claren-
241:1–3   don Press, 1930; Gavin de Beer, *Embryos and Ancestors.* 1st ed. 1940, 2nd ed. 1951, 3re ed. 1958.

:8–14   Ronald W. Clark, *JBS: The Life and Work of JBS Haldane.* New York: Coward-McCann, 1968.

241:8sq   J. B. S. Haldane, *The Causes of Evolution.* 2nd ed. London: Longmans, 1932.

:33–35   Yosiaki Itô, "Groups and Family Bonds in Animals in Relation to Their Habitats," in *Development and Evolution of Behavior,* Lester R. Aronson et al., (eds.), San Francisco: W. H. Freeman, 1970, p. 393.

:13–29   J. B. S. Haldane, "The Time of Action of Genes," *American*
:28 to   *Naturalist,* vol. 66, 1932, pp. 5–24.
242:1–21   J. B. S. Haldane, *The Causes of Evolution,* p. 124.

:34–39   J. B. S. Haldane, ibid., pp. 164–165.

243:1–8   Olaf Stapledon, *Last and First Men: A Story of the Near and Far Future.* London: Methuen, 1930.

:13–27   Julian S. Huxley, *Problems of Relative Growth.* New York: Lincoln MacVeagh, 1932, p. 239.

:32 to   Aldous Huxley, *After Many a Summer Dies the Swan.* London:
244:1–27   Chatto & Windus, 1939; New York: Harper & Brothers, 1939.

:4–6   Peter Bowering, *The Novels of Aldous Huxley.* London: The Athlone Press, 1968; Philip Thody, *Aldous Huxley: A Biographical Introduction.* New York: Scribner's, 1937.

:32–39   Frederic Wood Jones, "Man, Nature's Baby," in *Doctors in Shirtsleeves.* New York: Vista Press, 1940, pp. 86–109.

245:1–3   L. Cuénot, "L'Homme ce Néoténique," *Bulletin l'Académie Royale Belgique,* vol. 31, 1945, pp. 427–432; L. Cuénot, *Invention et Finalité en Biologie,* Paris, 1951; L. Cuénot, *L'Evolution Biologique.* Paris, 1951.

:3–7   Franck Bourdier, "Evolution Humaine et Juvénisme," *Bulletin de la Société Préhistorique Française,* No. 11–12, 1948, pp. 1–8.

:14sq   Gavin de Beer, "Embryology and the Evolution of Man," in *Robert Broom Commemorative Volume,* Alex L. Du Toit (ed.), Cape Town: Royal Society of South Africa, 1948, pp. 181–190.

:18–24   Gavin de Beer, ibid., p. 184.

:8–22   Gavin de Beer, "Peter Pan Evolution," 1951? Lost reference.

Page and line

:23 to   Gavin de Beer, "Paedomorphosis," *Proceedings of the XVth*
247:1–2   *International Congress of Zoology,* London, 1959, pp. 927–
         950, p. 930.

246:32–35   Gavin de Beer, *Embryos and Ancestors.* 3rd ed., Oxford: the
         Clarendon Press, 1958, p. 119.

247:3–16   Gavin de Beer, *Atlas of Evolution.* London and New York:
         Thomas Nelson, 1964, pp. 151–154.

:17–28   Ibid., p. 154.

247:33 to   Arnold Gehlen, *Der Mensch, seine Natur und seine Stellung in*
249:1–9   *der Welt.* Berlin: Athenaion, 1940/1975.

249:14 to   Konrad Lorenz, "Part and Parcel in Animal and Human
250:1–3   Societies." In Konrad Lorenz, *Studies in Animal and*
         Human Behaviour. vol. 2, Cambridge: Harvard University
         Press, 1971, pp. 115–195, p. 180.

250:24–30   Konrad Lorenz, ibid., p. 180.

:8 to   Weston La Barre, *The Human Animal.* Chicago: University of
251:1–2   Chicago Press, 1954.

:3–23   Weston La Barre, *The Ghost Dance.* New York: Doubleday,
         1970.

:15–23   Weston La Barre, ibid., p. 92.

:28 to   A. A. Abbie, "A New Approach to the Problem of Human
252:1–20   Evolution," *Transactions of the Royal Society of Austra-*
         lia. vol. 75, 1952, pp. 70–88, p. 84.

:26 to   George Gaylord Simpson, *Mode and Tempo in Evolution.* New
253:1–2   York: Columbia University Press, 1953.

:8–34   Ashley Montagu, "Time, Morphology, and Neoteny in the Evo-
         lution of Man," *American Anthropologist,* vol. 57, 1955, pp.
         13–17.

:34–37   Ashley Montagu, "Neoteny and the Evolution of the Hu-
         man Mind," *Explorations* (Toronto), no. 6, 1956, pp.
         85–90.

:37   Ashley Montagu, *Anthropology and Human Nature.* Boston:
         Porter Sargent, 1957.

:37   Ashley Montagu (ed.), *Culture and the Evolution of Man.* New
         York: Oxford University Press, 1962.

:38–39   Ashley Montagu, *The Human Revolution.* Cleveland & New
         York: World Publishing Co., 1965, pp. 167–183.

:38   Ashley Montagu, *An Introduction to Physical Anthropology.* 3rd
         ed. Springfield, Illinois: C C Thomas, 1960.

254:1–5   Theodosius Dobzhansky, *Mankind Evolving.* New Haven: Yale
         University Press, 1962, pp. 151 and 154.

:12–30   E. B. Ford and J. S. Huxley, "Mendelian Genes and Rates of
         Development in *Gammarus chevreuxi,*" *British Journal of*
         Experimental Biology, vol. 5, 1927, pp. 112–134.

:33–34   Julian Huxley, "The Evolutionary Process," in *Evolution as a*

Page and line

Process, J. S. Huxley, A. C. Hardy, and E. B. Ford (eds.). London: Allen & Unwin, 1954, p. 20.

:33–34   A. C. Hardy, "Escape from Specialization," in *Evolution as a Process,* J. S. Huxley, A. C. Hardy, and E. B. Ford (eds.). London: Allen & Unwin, 1954, p. 123.

255:1–19   Robert Kuttner, "An Hypothesis on the Evolution of Intelligence. *Psychological Reports,* vol. 6, 1960, pp. 283–289.

:24 to
257:1–20   R. F. Ewer, "Natural Selection and Neoteny," *Acta Biotheoretica,* vol. 13, 1960, pp. 161–184.

256:5   F. Kovács, "Biological Interpretation of the Nine-Month Duration of Human Pregnancy," *Acta Biologica Magyar,* vol. 10, 1960, pp. 331–361.

256:13–16   Le Gros Clark, W. E., *The Antecedents of Man.* 3rd ed. Chicago: Quadrangle Books, 1971, p. 22.

:17–22   C. Loring Brace and Ashley Montagu, *Human Evolution.* 2nd ed. New York: The Macmillan Company, 1977; E. M. B. Clements and S. Zuckerman, "The Order of Eruption of the Permanent Teeth in the Hominoidea," *American Journal of Physical Anthropology,* vol. 11, 1953, pp. 313–332; Albert A. Dahlberg, "Dental Evolution and Culture," *Human Biology,* vol. 35, 1963, pp. 237–249.

:32–39   Ewer, op. cit., p. 180.

257:36 to
258:1–3   Ernst Mayr, *Animal Species and Evolution.* Cambridge: Harvard University Press, 1963, p. 598.

:20 to
:1–28   William A. Mason, "Early Social Deprivation in the Nonhuman Primates: Implications for Human Behavior," in *Environmental Influences,* David C. Glass (ed.), New York: The Rockefeller University Press and Russell Sage Foundation, 1968, pp. 70–101.

:39 to   William A. Mason, ibid., 96.
259:1–3   William A. Mason, ibid., p. 100.
:24–28   William A. Mason, ibid., p. 101.

:33 to
260:1–23   David Jonas and Doris Klein, *Man-Child: A Study of the Infantilization of Man.* New York: McGraw-Hill, 1970, p. 339.

:19–18   Erik H. Erikson, *Childhood and Society,* 2nd ed. New York: W. W. Norton, 1963; Erik H. Erikson (ed.), *The Challenge of Youth.* New York: Anchor Books, 1963; John R. Gillis, *Youth and History.* New York: Academic Press, 1974; Paul Goodman, *Growing Up Absurd.* New York: Vintage Books, 1960; Christopher Lasch, *Haven in a Heartless World.* New York: Basic Books, 1977; Christopher Lasch, *The Culture of Narcissism.* New York: Norton, 1978.

:25 to
261:1–9   Robert B. Cairns, "The Ontogeny and Phylogeny of Social Interactions," in *Communicative Behavior and Evolution,*

Page and line

	Martin E. Hahn and Edward C. Simmel (eds.), New York: Academic Press, 1976, pp. 115–139.
:14–28	Roderic Gorney, *The Human Agenda*. New York: Simon & Schuster, 1972; reprinted Los Angeles: Guild of Tutors Press, 1979.
:27–28	Gorney, ibid., p. 557.
:33 to 262:1–30	R. Dale Guthrie, *Body Hot Spots: The Anatomy of Human Social Organs and Behavior*. New York: Van Nostrand Reinhold Co., 1976.
:35 to 263:1–34	Stephen Jay Gould, *Ontogeny and Phylogeny*. Cambridge: Harvard University Press, 1977.
263:11–17	Gould, ibid., p. 9.
:29–34	Stephen Jay Gould, "The Child as Man's Real Father," *Natural History*, vol. 84, 1975, pp. 18–22.
:32–34	Stephen Jay Gould, "Human Babies as Embryos," *Natural History*, vol. 85, 1976, pp. 22–26.
:34 to	Ashley Montagu, *An Introduction to Physical Anthropology*, 3rd. ed. Springfield, Illinois: C C Thomas, 1960, pp. 303–307.
264:3–5	Phillip V. Tobias (ed.), *The Bushmen: San Hunters and Herders of Southern Africa*. Cape Town & Pretoria: Human & Rousseau, 1978; Richard B. Lee and Irven DeVore (eds.), *Kalahari Hunter-Gatherers: Studies of !Kung San and Their Neighbors*. Cambridge: Harvard University Press, 1976; Lorna Marshall, *The !Kung of Nyae Nyae*. Cambridge: Harvard University Press, 1976; Richard B. Lee, *The !Kung San: Men, Women, and Work in a Foraging Society*. Cambridge: Harvard University Press, 1979; Richard B. Lee and Irven DeVore (eds.), *Man the Hunter*, Aldine Publishing Co., 1968; Marjorie Shostak, *Nisa: The Life and Words of a !Kung Woman*. Cambridge: Harvard University Press, 1981.
:23–26	Gavin de Beer, *Atlas of Evolution*. London & New York: Thomas Nelson, 1964, p. 153.

Index

About the Author

Ashley Montagu is one of the few experts on just about everything to do with people. He is, at last count, the author or editor of over sixty books on such varied subjects as anatomy and physiology, psychology, anthropology, race, evolution and heredity, love, aggression and touching, human development, sexuality, the history of science, the dangers of pollution, the anatomy of swearing, and the dolphin in human history. Among his classic works are *The Natural Superiority of Women, Man's Most Dangerous Myth: The Fallacy of Race, Human Evolution, The Elephant Man, Touching, Anthropology and Human Nature, Life Before Birth, On Being Human,* and *The Nature of Human Aggression.* He is co-author with Floyd Matson of *The Human Connection,* published by McGraw-Hill. He is the writer and director of the film "One World or None," described as one of the best documentaries ever made. Ashley Montagu teaches at Princeton University.